CONSUMER HEALTH

Second Edition

CONSUMER HEALTH

Second Edition

Kenneth L. Jones
Louis M. Shainberg
Curtis O. Byer

Mt. San Antonio College

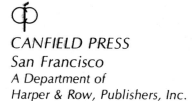

CANFIELD PRESS
San Francisco
A Department of
Harper & Row, Publishers, Inc.

CONSUMER HEALTH, Second Edition

Copyright © 1975 by Kenneth L. Jones, Louis W. Shainberg, and Curtis O. Byer

Library of Congress Cataloging in Publication Data:

Jones, Kenneth Lamar, 1931–
  Consumer health.

  Bibliography
  Includes index.

  1. Medical care—United States. 2. Medical care,
Cost of—United States. 3. Consumer protection—
United States. 4. Quacks and quackery—United
States.   I. Shainberg, Louis W., joint author.   II. Byer,
Curtis O., 1936– joint author.   III. Title   [DNLM:
1. Delivery of health care—U.S.—Popular works.
2. Economics, Medical—U.S. Popular works.   WB50 AA1 J7c]
RA410.53.J66   1975   362.1'0973   75-19062

ISBN 0-06-384369-2

Interior and cover design by Penny Faron

75   76   77   10   9   8   7   6   5   4   3   2   1

PREFACE

There is no doubt that Americans today attach high priority to living a long and disease-free life. People pay more for health services in this country than anywhere else in the world, indicating the importance we assign to good health. Freedom from pain and disease, through access to quality health services, is considered to be a basic human right, not a privilege of the wealthy. Unfortunately, the achievement of such a standard remains a clouded and uncertain hope for millions in our population. In the enlightened 1970s many people are bewildered as to whom they should seek out for health counsel; or if informed, are unable to locate the professional help they need; or having found help, are too poor to pay the professional fees asked. Physicians are not uniformly distributed; some hospitals in dense population clusters are over-crowded and understaffed. Adequate private health insurance is held by too few. The federal government's first attempts to provide national health care for selected high-need groups have been under-funded.

Because of consumer awareness, the public has begun to realize the need for and to demand improvements in both health products and services. With the leadership of active consumer groups and the response of government agencies, people realize that they no longer need to be the pawns of insensitive manufacturers. Pharmaceuticals, packaged foods, cosmetics, and toys are being improved due to consumer demand. Before the housecleaning is completed, health services as well as products may be deeply affected.

As if the selecting and financing of legitimate health products and services were not difficult enough, health charlatans (quacks) entice us with hundreds of questionable to worthless "remedies" at inflated prices. Far from being a thing of the past, today's quacks are often highly sophisticated in their newest schemes to dupe trusting clients. Virtually all of us fall prey to their efforts at one time or another.

The purpose of this book is to offer information concerning the selection of health services and products—physicians, cosmetics, food, drugs, hospitals, and health insurance plans. It is dedicated to helping people attain quality care and goods.

K.L.J.
L.W.S.
C.O.B.

CONTENTS

CONSUMER HEALTH

Second Edition

Chapter 1
THE CONSUMER
IN THE
MARKET PLACE

On January 1, 1975, a landmark regulation required by the federal Food and Drug Administration came into full effect. By that date food manufacturers had to comply with a new food labeling regulation called *nutrition labeling*. The manufacturer is required to list all ingredients and/or give a nutritional analysis of the food when he adds any nutrient or when he makes some nutritional claim on the label or in advertising.

This was just one of an increasing number of government actions, both federal and state, designed to develop accountability in the market place. Such actions are occurring with the active involvement of consumer groups nationwide. Consumers are becoming aware that their calls for responsibility in the delivery of products and services of many kinds are being heard. The strength of an active, unified consumer voice has been amply demonstrated. Without this voice, these changes would not be occurring. Consumers don't deserve all the credit, however. Effective action is the result of a balanced blend of participation by an enlightened government, a responsive producer of goods and services, as well as an active, discerning consumer.

Basic Rights of the Consumer

As early as 1962, President Kennedy stated four "basic rights" of the consumer:

> the right to safety;
> the right to be heard;
> the right to choose;
> the right to be informed.

During the past decade, consumer advocates have added a fifth right to this manifesto: the right to quality and integrity in the market place. These rights translate into obligations for consumers, as well as for businesspersons and government.

What is the nature of these obligations? It is the obligation of the consumer to be informed, to fully read advertisements and labels, to follow instructions, and to be aware of releases on consumer products and services in the public media. Consumers are obliged to make themselves heard. Those who believe they have been defrauded must notify and cooperate with authorities to prosecute the offender when the complaint is warranted.

Manufacturers and the providers of services are equally obligated. The businessperson is obliged to protect the health and safety of consumers in the design and manufacture of products and the provision of consumer services. This includes protection against side effects harmful to the quality of life and to the environment. It is their duty to seek out the informed view of consumers and other groups to help assure customer satisfaction from the earliest stages of product planning. They are responsible for eliminating fraud and deception from the market place, setting as a goal not merely strict legality, but honesty in all transactions. Their responsibilities also include providing consumers with objective information about products, services, and the workings of the market place through appropriate channels of communication, including programs of consumer education.

The government is responsible for the third side of this triangle of protection. Government is obliged to provide basic regulations and enforcement in product safety and effectiveness. As with nutrition labeling, it can be expected to demand comparative uniform labeling so the consumer retains the option of selecting the best value in quality and price. The government may also need to regulate the pricing of services to protect the consumer in those services where consumer selection is limited or absent.

Consumer Ignorance of Health Products

The Food and Drug Administration (FDA) recently conducted a national survey of consumers on foods, cosmetics, prescription drugs, nonprescription (over-the-counter) drugs, and toys. The data from the survey show that the majority of consumers (almost two-thirds of those questioned) are highly concerned about the safety of products they use in and around their homes. The majority believe that improper product usage is the most frequent cause of household accidents. These consumers believe that toys, drugs, and cosmetics are getting safer, while foods are getting less safe, although they still consider foods safer than any of the other categories surveyed. As to who does the most to make all types of products "as safe as they are," those surveyed suggest in order (a) the government, (b) consumer organizations, and (c) manufacturers of products. Most people recognize that the federal government is empowered to stop the sale of products that are found unsafe.

Consumers appeared to be less knowledgeable about the safety of drugs (medicines) than any of the other categories of products about which they were questioned. Answers to questions indicated a number of misconceptions about the relative safety of prescription drugs compared to over-the-counter (OTC) drugs. When asked to compare all categories in terms of safety, they ranked from safest to least safe in the following order: foods, prescription drugs, cosmetics, toys, and OTC drugs. Many were not quite sure why some OTC drugs are considered unsafe; about 15 percent felt that no OTC drugs should be purchased (although the FDA reviews them as to their safety and effectiveness).

Prescription drugs are felt to be safer because of consumer confidence in the physician. Yet there is the misconception that the government pretests drugs all or most of the time. Actually, the government pretests drugs only under certain circumstances. Every batch of antibiotics must be tested before marketing to assure proper potency. The government evaluates the safety and effectiveness of both prescription and nonprescription (OTC) drugs before they can be sold, but this evaluation is based on data submitted by manufacturers, not on government tests. Before the new drug is put on the market, the manufacturer must submit a New Drug Application to the FDA for complete review and approval. Included are data on studies as to the safety and effectiveness of the product, the chemicals and other materials used in the processing, and the conditions under which the drug will be manufactured. After approval is given, the manufacturer continues to batch-test the drug regularly. Once marketed, the drug is periodically sampled by the FDA to be sure it is meeting standards.

Another common misconception among consumers is that OTC drugs list all the ingredients in the product. Actually, by law manufacturers are required to list only the *active* ingredients of OTC drugs; inactive ingredients are listed only if the manufacturer chooses. The consumer is responsible for reading labels and following directions given therein.

Health Care Concerns

Nowhere is the need for consumer response and vigilance more apparent than in the field of health services and products. While products such as cosmetics and toys may relate to our enjoyment, they are really luxuries. Good health, on the other hand, is both a necessity and a basic human right. Quality services and products are essential to the maintenance of a person's health. Fraud in the field of health may mean not only loss of one's life savings but also disability. Lack of the services of a physician or the facilities of a hospital often affects our survival. What is the state of affairs in the delivery of health services and products in this country? Following is something of the picture.

Cost of Health Care

Many Americans fear the financial consequences of becoming seriously ill. For millions, going to the hospital means going broke or close to it. For many more, good medical care is nonexistent. Underlining the cost of disease to this country is the fact that the total health bill for Americans now stands at over $82 billion a year. This represents nearly 8 percent of our gross national product (a greater proportion for health care than in any other country), or better than $350 per person per year.

As medical techniques have improved, fewer people are dying from certain maladies; however, this is being accomplished at rapidly rising costs. A study from Massachusetts General Hospital is a case in point. It is a comparison of patients coming to the hospital with coronary occlusions (heart attacks), in terms of cost per patient and fatalities, for the years 1920, 1940, and 1970:

Year	Patients	Fatalities	Cost per Patient
1920	100	40	$200
1940	100	30	$400-600
1970	100	16	$3500

Thus, although the number of fatalities from coronary occlusions has been reduced, this reduction has been achieved at great cost.

In 1972, personal expenditures for health care exceeded $21 billion, or two and a half times what they were in 1962. For the same period, the amount spent for all personal items doubled. In other words, while a person spent 5.6 percent of his disposable (spendable) income for health care in 1962, he spent 7.0 percent in 1972.

In spite of past increases in health costs, all indications point to even higher costs, if the delivery of health services is to be improved to any extent. Some are even predicting that by 1980 hospital costs for intensive care may rise to at least $1,000 per day per bed. Already, costs in excess of $100 per day per bed are average, with intensive care now averaging $300 to $500 per day.

Regardless of such costs, gaps still exist in the percentage of the population covered by private health insurance. Although public health insurance is available to those age 65 and over, most persons under 65 desiring insured health services must seek coverage from private insurance companies. Sixteen million Americans under sixty-five, or 8 percent of the population, have no health insurance at all.

How Americans Rank Worldwide

Unfortunately, even with this great expenditure of money, the United States has been falling behind other nations in such key areas as infant mortality and life expectancy. In infant mortality we presently rank 20th (Table 1.1). In the number of years adults live, we rank 24th worldwide (Table 1.2). Sweden, by contrast, spends only 5 percent of her gross national product on health services and stands relatively high in both tables.

TABLE 1.1. Infant Mortality per Country

Rank	Country	Infant Mortality per 1000 Births
1	Finland	10
2	Sweden	10
3	Iceland	12
4	Japan	12
5	Netherlands	12
6	Norway	13
7	Switzerland	13
8	Denmark	14
9	Spain	15
10	France	16
11	Luxembourg	16
12	New Zealand	16
13	Australia	17
14	Belgium	17
15	Canada	17
16	Hong Kong	17
17	East Germany	18
18	Ireland	18
19	United Kingdom	18
20	United States	18
21	Singapore	20
22	West Germany	20
23	Czechoslovakia	21
24	Israel	21
25	Austria	24

Source: *1975 World Population Data Sheet*, Population Reference Bureau, Inc., Washington, D.C., 1975.

TABLE 1.2. Life Expectancy per Country

Rank	Country	Life Expectancy at Birth
1	Iceland	74
2	Netherlands	74
3	Norway	74
4	Belgium	73
5	East Germany	73
6	France	73
7	Japan	73
8	Sweden	73
9	Australia	72
10	Bulgaria	72
11	Canada	72
12	Greece	72
13	Ireland	72
14	Italy	72
15	New Zealand	72
16	Puerto Rico	72
17	Spain	72
18	Switzerland	72
19	United Kingdom	72
20	Austria	71
21	Cyprus	71
22	Israel	71
23	Luxembourg	71
24	United States	71
25	West Germany	71

Source: 1975 World Population Data Sheet, Population Reference Bureau, Inc., Washington, D.C., 1975.

Loss of Productivity

Americans lose millions of days from work every year due to acute illnesses and injuries which last less than three months and which involve either medical attention or restricted activity. In 1971, according to the United States National Health Survey, wage earners lost over 262 million work days as a result of some acute condition. This amounted to an average of 3.4 days off the job per worker.

Injuries resulted in an average of 1.0 work days lost per person per year. The survey showed that home accidents were the most frequent single cause of injury, followed in order by injuries from motor vehicles and at work.

This survey reflected a distinct difference in days of disability between the low and middle income brackets. The average American had 16 days of restricted activity as a result of an acute and/or chronic condition. The average number of bed-disability days was 6, while the average number of work-loss days was 5. Persons from families with an annual income of less than $3,000 averaged 34 restricted activity days, while those from families with an income of $10,000 to $14,999 had an average of 12 days (Table 1.3). Average bed-disability days for the less than $3,000 income group was 12½, while the average for the $10,000–$14,999 class was 4½ days. Those with incomes under $3,000 had an annual average of 9 days away from the job, while in the $10,000–$14,999 bracket, workers averaged 4½ work-loss days.

Major Causes of Death in the United States

The effects of disease have changed significantly during the past seventy years. The major causes of death in the United States at the turn of the century and in 1972 are compared in Table 1.4.

The causes of death differ at different ages in life. Accidents top the list from childhood through age forty-five. The five leading causes of death, arranged by age group and ranked from one (most frequent) through five, are:

1. *Infant mortality* (under 1 year of age). (1) congenital malformations, (2) postnatal asphyxia, (3) premature birth, (4) influenza and pneumonia, and (5) birth injuries.

2. *Preschool children* (ages 1 through 4). (1) accidents, (2) influenza and pneumonia, (3) congenital malformations, (4) cancers, and (5) meningitis.

3. *Elementary and junior high school students* (ages 5 through 14). (1) accidents, (2) cancers, (3) congenital malformations, (4) influenza and pneumonia, and (5) heart diseases.

4. *Senior high school and college-age persons* (ages 15 through 24). (1) accidents, (2) homicide, (3) suicide, (4) cancers, and (5) heart diseases.

5. *Young adults and parents* (ages 25 through 44). (1) accidents, (2) heart diseases, (3) cancers, (4) homicide, and (5) suicide.

6. *Middle-aged persons* (ages 45 through 64). (1) heart diseases, (2) cancers, (3) stroke, (4) accidents, and (5) cirrhosis of the liver.

7. *The elderly* (ages 65 and over). (1) heart diseases, (2) cancers, (3) stroke, (4) influenza and pneumonia, and (5) hardening of the arteries.

The leading killer diseases are heart diseases and cancers. Over 52 percent of all deaths among all ages in the United States are due to the effects of the cardiovascular diseases (heart, cerebral hemorrhage, and other vascular causes); 18 percent due to cancers and other malig-

TABLE 1.3. Disability Days by Family Income and Type of Disability (in the United States, 1971)

Type of Disability	All Incomes	Under $3,000	$3,000– $4,999	$5,000– $6,999	$7,000– $9,999	$10,000– $14,999	$15,000 and Over
				Family Income			
Restricted Activity							
Days (000,000 omitted)	3176	665	439	414	479	573	402
Days per person per year	15.7	33.7	20.7	15.3	12.8	11.8	11.3
Bed Disability							
Days (000,000 omitted)	1239	249	178	155	186	226	160
Days per person per year	6.1	12.6	8.4	5.7	5.0	4.6	4.5
Work-Loss Days							
Days (000,000 omitted)	396	41	42	57	74	93	65
Days per person per year	5.1	9.4	6.6	5.7	5.0	4.5	4.0

Note: The data refer to disability because of acute and/or chronic conditions. The category "All incomes" includes unknown income. The category "Work-Loss Days" applies to currently employed persons.

Source: National Health Survey, U.S. Department of Health, Education, and Welfare.

TABLE 1.4. Causes of Death in the United States

Order	1900	1972
1	Influenza and pneumonia	Heart diseases
2	Tuberculosis	Cancers
3	Gastroenteritis	Stroke
4	Heart diseases	All accidents
5	Stroke	Influenza and pneumonia
6	Chronic nephritis	Diabetes mellitus
7	All accidents	Cirrhosis of liver
8	Cancers	Hardening of arteries
9	Diseases of early infancy	Diseases of early infancy
10	Diphtheria	Bronchitis, emphysema, and asthma

Source: *Monthly Vital Statistics Report, Provisional Statistics, Annual Summary for U.S.*, 1973, Vol. 22, No. 13, June 27, 1974.

nant growths; and 6 percent due to accidents. (In 1900, these causes were responsible for all deaths in the United States in this proportion; cardio-vascular diseases, 14 percent; cancers and other malignant growths, 4 percent; and accidents, 4 percent.) It is estimated that one adult in four can anticipate developing a fatal heart ailment; one in every four can expect to suffer from cancer. While two out of every three cancer victims die, many of these die needlessly. Today well-established cancer-detection methods are ignored by many adults.

Improvements During the Next Decade

What about the near future? Look for improvements during the next ten years in these areas of health services:

1. Services more available and accessible to those most in need.

2. Services which stress health education, disease prevention, rehabilitation, earlier diagnosis, and improved treatment.

3. An improved system of insurance coverage for the great majority of the population against medical expenses, either through private insurance or a national health insurance program.

4. Improvements in efficient hospital management and better systems for keeping physicians' fees within reasonable limits.

But these developments are still in the future. How can a person get best use out of the available dollars he has to spend for health service now? The following chapters are written to provide some guidance.

Summary

I. Consumer Voice Being Heard by Both Government and Business

II. Basic Rights of the Consumer

    A. Right to safety

    B. Right to be heard

    C. Right to choose

    D. Right to be informed

    E. Right to quality and integrity in the market place

III. Consumer Ignorance of Health Products

    A. Less knowledge of drugs than of toys and cosmetics

    B. Consumer distrust of nonprescription (over-the-counter) drugs

    C. Consumer misconceptions on drugs:

        1. That the government pretests drugs all or most of the time

        2. That nonprescription drugs must list all the ingredients in the product

IV. Health Care Concerns

    A. Cost of Health Care

        1. Health care costs $350 per person per year

        2. Personal expenditures for health care in 1972 were 2½ times what they were in 1962, compared with a doubling of all personal expenses

        3. Eight percent of all Americans have no health insurance of any kind

    B. How Americans Rank Worldwide

        1. In infant mortality we rank 20th

        2. In longevity we rank 24th

    C. Loss of Productivity

        1. Average American loses 3.4 work days per year due to some acute condition

        2. Injuries result in average of 1.0 lost work days per person per year

        3. Those with family incomes of less than $3,000 per year averaged 34 restricted activity days for acute/chronic conditions, while those from family incomes of $10,000 to $14,999 averaged 12 days of restricted activity

    D. Major Causes of Death in the United States

        1. Top causes of death in 1900 were (in order) influenza and pneumonia, tuberculosis, gastroenteritis, heart diseases, and stroke

2. Top causes of death in 1972 were (in order) heart diseases, cancers, stroke, accidents, and influenza/pneumonia

3. Over 70 percent of all deaths in the United States among all ages are due to heart diseases and cancers

E. Improvements During the Next Decade

1. More available and accessible services to those in need

2. Improved health education, disease prevention, rehabilitation, earlier diagnosis, and improved treatment

3. Population-wide national health insurance program

4. Greater efficiency in hospital management and better control over physicians' fees

Questions for Review

1. List the five basic rights of consumers.

2. What are the obligations of consumers, businesspersons, and government in obtaining quality and integrity for consumers in the market place?

3. Compare government testing and approval for antibiotics, other prescription drugs, and nonprescription drugs.

4. The cost per patient for treatment of certain maladies has risen significantly during the past fifty years. How does such increase relate to reduction in fatalities?

5. How do increases in money spent for health care during the past ten years compare with money spent for all personal items?

6. Compare Sweden and the United States in infant mortality and longevity for adults.

7. Americans experience many days of restricted activity or work loss each year. How does loss of productivity relate to level of income?

8. Where did the five top causes of death in the United States for 1972 stand in 1900?

9. Trace the position of heart diseases as a cause of death among the various age groups. Do the same for cancers.

10. List the improvements in health services that are anticipated during the coming decade.

Chapter 2

CHOOSING
MEDICAL
SERVICES

Medicine has made unbelievable advancements within the past century. During the past fifteen years vaccines have been developed for poliomyelitis, measles, and rubella (German measles). Research is making a massive assault on the causes of and cures for cancer. Mental retardation, once considered an unpreventable malady, is now known to have various causes, some of which are preventable. Many diseases are so well controlled today that we give little or no thought to them; the causes and cures of others will, without doubt, be discovered within the next decade. The importance of all this is that a child born today can anticipate a life expectancy half again as long as his ancestors could fifty years ago.

Such medical benefits come to us as much through readily available medical care as through work in the research laboratory. But wanting the best in medical care and getting it may be two different matters. It becomes essential for a person to know how to choose medical care.

Modern Medicine

Goals

The hopes of medicine today can best be expressed in four major objectives:

1. Good medical care must be available to *all* people, both the financially comfortable and the economically deprived.

2. The *prevention,* as much as the cure, of disease must be given top priority.

3. The needs of the *whole person* must be cared for. The specialties and subspecialties treat only parts of the person rather than viewing him as an integrated individual.

4. Research into unconquered diseases and improved methods of treatment must be well funded.

While none of these objectives have yet been realized, they continue to guide the medical profession.

Problems Faced by Today's Physician

In spite of the depth of their training and their rank in the community, there are some pressing problems facing physicians. One such problem is the increasing shortage of physicians. Due to population increases, it is estimated that the current shortage of physicians in the United States is about 50,000. Rather than improving, the shortage is getting worse. Just 60 years ago there was one physician for every 568 persons in the U.S.; by a recent census, there is now one for every 804 persons. (Such ratios are still mild compared to some Third World countries which have one physician for every 25,000 to 30,000 persons.) Compounding this shortage is the increasing demand the public is making on physicians' services. Today the average American sees a physician five times a year, twice as often as he did in 1930.

Available physicians are not evenly distributed throughout the population. The physician-patient ratio is more favorable in urban areas than in rural ones. Some physicians prefer to practice in urban locations, which offer better hospitals, higher incomes, and more cultural advantages for their families. The upshot of such concentration is that scattered rural communities may have few or no physicians.

Not all physicians are available for family health care. The majority of physicians prefer to restrict their practice to a specialized area of medicine, due in part to the desire to be competent practitioners. One bright spot in this picture is the inception of the new medical specialty of Family Practice (discussed later in this chapter).

The image the public has of the medical profession is also changing. As medical care has become more mechanized, as more duties are relegated to medical aides and paramedicals, and as his or her time has been placed in greater demand, the physician doesn't always take time to explain things well enough to patients. Many patients are well-read and informed and want to know the nature of their ailments. They are prepared to accept a little less personal attention if they have some idea of what is going on.

While the physician has been professionally trained to communicate in concise technical terms, he or she must be prepared to describe things in a language the layman understands.

Medical costs have risen faster during the past two decades than increases in other personal expenditures. Although an analysis shows that some of these higher costs are the direct results of higher hospital costs and improved methods of diagnosis and therapy, the public tends to place the blame for higher medical costs on physicians. Given the choice between health and illness or death, however, most patients prefer the better, albeit costlier, treatment. Yet it is imperative that the rising costs of health care not get out of reach of people, preventing some from receiving adequate care.

Changes in Medical Practice

In the last forty years, general practitioners have dropped from 74 percent to 16 percent of all physicians in the country. Medical students have viewed the GP as a "nice guy, but not terribly well trained." Yet these same students are increasingly unhappy with the narrow specialties that treat only a particular disease or organ, and the tide is now turning in favor of general practice. The new Family Practice specialty is preparing the specialist in general medicine. There is also strong interest in the specialties of internal medicine and pediatrics.

There is widespread feeling politically and medically that health insurance must be made available to all people. Such insurance is as essential for low income families as Medicare/Medicaid was for the elderly, if these families are to be provided basic health care. Where business and industry are too slow in providing sufficient, reasonably priced insurance coverage, the federal and state governments have started stepping in. The result is that the percentage of Americans covered by some form of health insurance has been increasing (Fig. 6.3).

The patterns of medical practice have been changing. More physicians are banding together into group practices in which certain services are shared (buildings, nursing and clerical services, laboratory). Such group practice models are particularly important in more remote rural areas. More physicians are moving into suburban and rural vicinities and creating their own hospital-like services by uniting into medical groups or clinics. There is increasing use of clinics and outpatient (ambulatory) services by general hospitals due to the centralized facilities available in many hospitals. These changes are helping improve the delivery of comprehensive health care services.

Choosing a Physician

The informed person knows that it is impossible for people to maintain good health apart from qualified medical counsel. But there are many different kinds of physicians, and perplexing questions still face many people: "What type of a physician would be the ideal medical adviser for my situation, and how do I find him?" Before these questions can be adequately answered, it is necessary to become acquainted with the training required of each type of medical practitioner.

Requirements to Practice

Before being licensed to practice medicine, one must meet certain professional and ethical requirements. Although training standards vary somewhat from state to state, three to four years of premedical college work are required. The prospective physician must then complete a four-year training program in a medical school approved by the Association of American Medical Colleges and the Council on Medical Education of the American Medical Association. In addition, most states require a one-year hospital internship following medical school. Before being allowed to practice in a given state, a physician must be licensed by a board of medical examiners. This license is granted only after the physician has passed either a state or a national board examination, depending upon the particular state. In addition to these basic requirements, if a physician desires to take a residency in a hospital to receive advanced training, or to meet the requirements for a given specialty in medicine, he or she must spend additional years (two to five) in training.

Standards for the training of physicians, as well as the ethics of medical practice, are set by the medical profession itself. The medical profession also assumes the responsibility for regulating the professional conduct and ethics of its members. Much of this regulation is handled through local and county medical societies. Most of these societies have adopted standards for their members, such as prohibiting advertising, refraining from guaranteeing cures, adhering to all legalities regarding the taking of human life and the administration of drugs, cooperating with legal authorities, and giving evidence of their trustworthiness through all public and private contacts. Not all physicians meet all such standards. In this respect, physicians, as a whole, are no different from any other professional group. In choosing a physician, we should have both the privilege and right of being satisfied both with his reputation, private and public, and with his professional qualifications. To the physician we entrust our lives.

A Family Physician

Everyone should have a personal or family physician. This physician should have a basic medical history of the patient and should provide for general comprehensive medical care. The family physician should refer the patient to the services of medical specialists if and when required. Such general family care is usually provided by the general practitioner, the family practitioner, or the general internist.

General Practitioner (GP)

In the past, many Americans looked almost solely to a single physician to diagnose and treat all the family's illnesses. The physician practiced general medicine and attempted to handle the full range of health conditions. In 1931, 74 percent of the physicians in the country were GPs; by the end of 1970 only 16 percent of all physicians were GPs.

Physicians are entitled to practice general medicine after they have completed medical school training, served one year of internship in general hospital practice, and passed the state or national board examinations required for licensure in that particular state. Although not required, most recent graduates take additional, or postgraduate, training of some kind. Today many practicing GPs have completed at least two years of residency training.

Some unique problems face the general practitioner today. In order to maintain a high-quality practice, the GP must keep abreast of the mass of new medical information and changes in medical techniques. This problem has led to a new medical specialty, Family Practice.

Family Practice

The need for a better trained physician who can give patients long-term comprehensive care led to the creation of this specialty in 1969. Graduate training programs are longer (three or four years), more specific, and more comprehensive than the GP graduate programs. The training varies somewhat from one hospital to another. Some programs emphasize internal medicine, psychiatry, and surgery, whereas others stress obstetrics and pediatrics. Upon completion of the hospital residency, the physician must pass a board examination given by the American Academy of Family Practice. The main concern with Family Practice is getting to know the family, rather than concern with a particular disease or organ, as in Internal Medicine. Thus, the main goal of Family Practice is to turn out physicians who can take care of most of the patient-family illnesses and injuries. In rural areas, the general practitioner's problem of keeping abreast of new medical developments and maintaining professional competence is being solved with the formation of group family practice model units. These model units are publicly funded experiments in groups of Family Practice specialists practicing together in a clinical group, yet maintaining close contact with the continuing educational programs of large nearby hospitals.

General Internist

The specialist in internal medicine may or may not fill the role of family physician. Such a specialist is generally better qualified to serve as a personal physician to adults rather than to children. An internist must have completed three years of training in an approved hospital after medical school and passed the examination given by the American Board of Internal Medicine. Since the training is primarily in diagnosis, the internist is particularly suited for preventive medicine, as well as for coordinating the work of specialists needed to treat the specific problems the patient faces. Not all internists desire to practice general medicine; some confine their work to subspecialties such as allergy, heart disease, digestive-tract problems, or lung ailments. Generally, internists do not deliver babies, practice surgery, deal with eye diseases or refractory corrections, or treat children.

The Specialties

The more physicians concentrate their attention on a given system of the body, the less time they have for the whole person and the less proficient they are in general practice. To thoroughly know one area of medicine, physicians must confine themselves to it to the exclusion of other areas. Such concentration has been necessary in order for medicine to make its great strides in heart surgery, cancer treatment and prevention, psychiatry, orthopedics, surgery, and other areas. Usually a recognized specialist must have completed a hospital residency of three to four years beyond formal medical training and passed the written examination required for that particular specialty. The physician is then recognized as a *board diplomate* of that particular specialty (such as, Diplomate of the American Board of Psychiatry).

Brief descriptions of several fields of specialization are given below.

Internal Medicine

Although internal medicine often deals with the total person, the practice of internal medicine is recognized as one of the specialties. The characteristics of that specialty have already been described.

Obstetrics and Gynecology

Obstetrics is the care of the woman in pregnancy and childbirth. It is frequently combined with gynecology (the care of women's diseases). Stressing preventive medicine, the obstetrician sees the mother early in pregnancy, supervises her health, and handles the delivery. Such attention has reduced infant mortality in this country and assures the best possible health for both the child and the mother.

Pediatrics

Pediatricians specialize in the care of infants and children. They advise parents, give checkups, diagnose congenital deformities, administer immunizations, and treat childhood diseases. Some pediatricians confine themselves to certain types of children's illnesses, such as cardiovascular disorders or pediatric allergies.

Surgery

The work of the surgeon involves surgically operating upon the patient to correct some physical condition. It may involve removing a cancer, repairing a defective heart, setting a broken bone, or attempting to correct a damaged brain. Since the body is so intricate, this specialty is subdivided into specific areas such as neurosurgery, thoracic surgery, orthopedic surgery, and abdominal surgery.

Psychiatry

Psychiatry deals with emotional illnesses and disturbances and mental retardation through the use of counseling and/or psychotherapy, as well as through the use of drugs, surgery, convulsive therapy, (treatment in which electric current, insulin, carbon dioxide, or metrazol is administered to the patient and results in a convulsive reaction to alter favorably the course of illness), and hydrotherapy. The psychiatrist is a medical specialist who holds an M.D. degree; some are also specialists in neurology. By distinction, a psychologist generally holds a graduate Ph.D. or M.A. degree (nonmedical degrees) and may engage in experimental, teaching, or clinical work. The clinical psychologist usually has further training in a medical setting and diagnoses and treats emotional and neurological disorders by the use of psychological methods rather than by medical measures. (By contrast, a counselor could be anyone giving advice to people with problems.) Any psychologist or psychiatrist using counseling or psychoanalytical methods in dealing with patients is also recognized as a psychotherapist.

Pathology

Pathology is the study of the disease process. Being concerned with the nature of disease, the pathologist looks for the structural and functional changes in tissues and organs of the body and identifies the disease causing the change, such as cancer. Some are employed by hospitals, while others have their own private practices. They also perform autopsies, and some serve as coroners.

Other fields of medical specialty include:

1. Anesthesiology, administering general and local anesthetics.
2. Dermatology, treating diseases of the skin.
3. Neurology, dealing with physical diseases of the brain and nervous system.
4. Ophthalmology, treating the eye and its diseases.
5. Otolaryngology, treating diseases of the ear, nose, and throat.
6. Proctology, treating diseases of the rectum and anus.
7. Radiology, using x-rays, radium, and other radioactive sources for the diagnosis and treatment of disease.

8. Urology, treating diseases and abnormalities of the urinary tract in the female and urinary and genital (urogenital) tract in the male.

9. Emergency Medicine, the newest specialty: the administering of emergency medical procedures of all kinds; practice is usually confined to the emergency room of a hospital.

There are over thirty recognized fields of medical specialization today. Each is governed by its respective board for purposes of examination and certification.

Osteopathy

Osteopathy is considered another field of medicine, and those trained in it are referred to as physicians.

It may be interesting to know why there are two similar fields of medical practice in this country. Around 1870 a physician named Dr. Andrew Still held that disease could be based on disturbed nerve functions which result from a pinching of the nerves as they leave the spinal column. According to this theory, a disease or condition in any particular organ of the body could be traced to a lesion in the nerve supplying that organ.

The medical profession has considered this theory unfounded and contradictory to its knowledge of human anatomy and pathology. Over the course of years, however, osteopathic physicians have been quietly abandoning many of the peculiar tenets originally held in osteopathy and have increasingly emphasized the place of drugs in the practice of sound medicine. This change has progressed to such an extent that today their training and practice is similar to that of traditional medical doctors, but with more emphasis on musculo-skeletal manipulation. Nonetheless, osteopaths are usually barred from practicing in medical hospitals.

Depending on the state in which a person resides, he or she will have greater or lesser interest in osteopathy. Moves have been initiated in various state medical societies to unite the medical and osteopathic professions, but only one has been accomplished so far. In 1962 California, recognizing that the quality of osteopathic training was closely similar to that of medicine, passed legislation enabling osteopaths in that state to be henceforth considered as M.D.'s. All former osteopathic colleges in California now bestow the M.D. degree upon their graduates. Significantly, this move came about as the result of a joint effort between osteopathic and medical societies within that state.

Some families prefer the services of an osteopathic physician. A qualified osteopath can satisfactorily serve as a family physician.

Types of Practice

It has been very common in the past for physicians to practice as individuals, located in isolated, single-person offices. Many physicians, particularly in more rural areas, still tend to practice in this manner. In recent years, however, physicians have increasingly favored banding together in various kinds of groups to provide better care than they could give in solo practices. Although the clinic has been commonly used for years in larger medical centers, such as the Mayo Clinic in Rochester, Minnesota, the average local physician practiced independently prior to World War II. Since 1946 the number of medical groups and the number of physicians in groups have both tripled. Various types of group practices can now be found in virtually every community.

Group practices tend to represent more than the simple sharing of facilities. Medical groups may consist of physicians in general practice or physicians from different specialties uniting with the idea of giving complete medical care to their patients. The majority of them include fewer than six physicians. Since the physicians work to some extent as a team, this arrangement allows for more frequent consultation and less inconvenience to the patient in making and keeping appointments.

Selecting the Right Physician

In selecting medical care, one must determine personal and family need and then find out what is available. Some people prefer a general practitioner, while others choose several specialists in selected branches of medicine. Since some general practitioners restrict themselves to a narrow branch of practice, it is necessary to know the nature of a physician's practice. If the family includes young children, the physician chosen should be one who enjoys working with children. The same point applies with elderly people. A person who cannot find one ideal physician for the entire family may prefer settling for several specialists, such as a pediatrician for the children and an internist for the adults.

In selecting a physician, either for general practice or to deal with a specific problem, there are certain procedures worth following that can help guarantee that you will find a physician well suited to your needs and temperament.

1. Consider the reputation of various physicians in your community. Contact a local *accredited* hospital for the names and addresses of the physicians who practice through that hospital. There is usually a relationship between the quality of a hospital and the quality of the physician who practices there.

You may wish to look into the educational credentials of a particular physician. These are known to the local or county medical society, by the local hospital in which he or she practices, or are listed in the *AMA Directory* or in *The Directory of Medical Specialists*. These will tell you whether the physician is licensed to practice in your state, where he or she has taken basic medical training, and where and when he or she has taken postgraduate work. These books may be found in some public libraries or in a hospital library.

If you are considering physicians who have been recommended by friends and relatives, you should be prepared to do some independent investigating. Other people's attitudes toward their physicians and their own illnesses might not be useful to you. It is wise, however, to stay away from physicians who consistently cause dissatisfaction among people whose judgment you respect.

2. Visit the office of the physician you are considering. The office should be within easy commuting distance. Find out if the physician is accepting new patients and if the office is neat, clean, and orderly. You may wish to set up an appointment with the physician. Since you are using the physician's professional time, you should plan on paying the fee for the usual office call. Discuss with the physician such topics as provision of general medical care for you or your family, his or her availability for house calls and emergencies, other physicians who can provide these services in the event he or she is out of town, and the fee schedule and how it compares with that of other physicians in town.

He or she should be a person in whom you can confide and who appears interested in your family's health and well-being. If you are satisfied regarding these points, you have found your physician.

The Patient–Physician Relationship

The patient is entitled to receive careful, professional service from the physician, including laboratory test results and consultations with any medical specialists necessary for adequate medical treatment. It may not always be possible for the physician to cure, but the patient should always have reason to feel that the physician is doing his best.

The physician should be as concerned with preventing disease as with curing it. Patients should be kept well-informed as to when inoculations and periodic examinations should be given. In the practice of *preventive* medicine it may be difficult for patients to understand the full benefit of medical care and justify the cost of it. Prevention of illness is not only easier, but less painful, cheaper and less time consuming. A careful physician would much rather prevent illness than attempt to bring an ailing patient back to health.

The patient should understand the physician's fee schedule. If the cost of medical care is imposing a genuine hardship on the patient or the family, the physician will want to know about it. The physician may be willing to adjust fees in the case of hardship. The patient should feel no embarrassment in raising such a discussion.

In return, the physician may expect certain courtesies from the patient. In nonemergencies the patient should make appointments and then *keep* them punctually. Medical bills should be paid as soon as possible. The patient should follow the physician's instructions exactly. If medication is prescribed it should be purchased immediately and taken as directed. The physician has a right to expect the confidence of patients.

A physician is not necessarily under obligation to answer emergency calls from unknown individuals late at night in the caller's home. The physician will have no medical history on the patient and may be subjecting himself to physical hazard or fatigue. Some individuals moving into a new community may fail to contact a new physician until they need one in emergency or late at night. Then, if difficulty in obtaining care is encountered, they make complaints against the medical profession. In such an emergency, the nearest *general* hospital should have physicians on duty who can provide care.

Physicians can give their best service when they feel that patients appreciate their efforts. As much as they would enjoy being able to cure every physical ailment, medical research has not provided them with all the necessary answers to accomplish this aim. But a good physician will go just as far in diagnosis and treatment as his or her ability, training, available facilities, and patients allow.

Chiropractic

It is necessary to make some mention and clarification of chiropractic. This profession is a system of treatment based on the belief that the nervous system largely determines a person's state of health and that any interference with this system impairs normal functions and lowers the body's resistance to disease. Patients are treated primarily by specific adjustment of parts of the body, especially the spinal column. X-ray is used extensively to aid in locating the source of the difficulty. Supplementary-treatment measures such as diet, exercise, rest, water, light, and heat are used. Chiropractic treatment by law cannot include the use of drugs or surgery. The training of chiropractors, although ranging from two to four years, consists in most states of four years of training in a chiropractic school following high school or one to two years of college work. Graduation does not qualify a chiropractor to practice in all states, since not all states license the practice of chiropractic.

Since many of the body's ailments are due to infections or degenerative diseases, any field of the healing arts that does not qualify a practitioner in the diagnosis and treatment of these kinds of maladies is restricted in usefulness. Most chiropractors are better trained in body manipulation and adjustment than they are in adequate understanding and diagnosis of the underlying disease. As interpreters of x-rays, their qualifications are not to be confused with the radiologist, a medical specialist. The academic and professional training beyond high school for the chiropractor may be six years, whereas it is twelve years for a radiologist (who also holds an M.D. degree). A check of the catalogues of chiropractic schools, which list names and degrees of faculty, shows that significant numbers of their faculty do not have generally recognized college degrees. Nor are their colleges accredited by the recognized educational bodies that accredit institutions of higher learning in the United States. Consequently, although the chiropractor may bring relief to conditions where the spinal column or a joint are maladjusted, there are many common medical conditions he is not prepared to care for. The chiropractor is not a medical doctor and should not be sought out as a family physician. It is the official position of the American Medical Association that "chiropractic is an unscientific cult whose practitioners lack the necessary training and background to diagnose and treat human disease." As a theory it fails to follow the scientific method of the making and testing of hypotheses, and the publishing of results so that others can repeat the same experiment in order to confirm or correct the original conclusions.

Dentistry

Dental training consists of four years of professional training following two to four years of required college work. A dental specialty usually requires two or three years of additional professional training. The majority of dentists are general practitioners who provide many types of dental care. If an individual is in need of a dental specialist, a general dentist will be more than glad to recommend one who will provide the required treatment.

Although there has been an actual increase in the number of dentists in the United States, the number has not kept pace with the increasing population. Since 1950 there has been a 34 percent increase in dentists, but this has resulted in a 1 percent actual *decrease* compared to the population.

Nursing

The nursing team is led by the professional or *registered nurse* (R.N.) but also includes the vocational nurse, nursing aide, medical technologist, orderly, and attendant. Registered nursing training requires two to four years of professional training beyond high school. Additional training can be taken to qualify a nurse in a nursing specialty (such as obstetrics, pediatrics, psychiatry, or surgical nursing).

Since 1960 the number of nurses has increased 61 percent. About 29 percent of all professional nurses work on a part-time basis. Also, the number of male nurses is increasing, and today males account for one percent of all professional nurses.

Facilities for Patient Care

As medical techniques have improved, so have facilities for patient care. Today's physician makes few home visits, particularly in urban areas. The home usually no longer serves as a "hospital" for delivery of babies, treatment of tuberculosis and pneumonia, or nursing home for elderly people suffering from chronic diseases. Today only minor illnesses are cared for at home. Improved standards of diagnosis and treatment require facilities available only in physicians' offices, clinics, nursing homes, and hospitals.

Nursing Homes

Providing health services for patients who are convalescent, chronically ill, or elderly is the function of nursing homes. Care here is less intensive as well as less expensive than that of a hospital. Developed as a result of the 1935 Social Security Act, private nursing homes have become both numerous and profitable. Later the Act was amended to also provide for care in public nursing homes.

Although many of the more than 13,000 nursing homes in the country provide excellent care, it is important that one be aware of wide differences in care when making a selection. One assurance of quality is accreditation of the home by the Joint Commission on Accreditation of Hospitals. Granted on a yearly basis, such accreditation assures that certain standards are being met, such as adequate fire and safety precautions, cleanliness of patient care, accurate and up to date records, a staff dietician, menu planning and food storage, and a planned activities program. Beyond such assurances, an individual should check fee rates, proximity, and available openings.

Hospitals

Population increases, along with greater physician use of hospitals, have substantially increased public demand for hospital facilities. Today there are more than 7000 hospitals of all kinds in the United States.

Kinds of Hospitals

Hospitals may be either public or private. Some provide medical care of all kinds, while others offer selected medical services to certain groups of people. Generally, hospitals can be grouped according to type of ownership and basis of receiving support.

Government Hospitals

Federal government hospitals have been established for military personnel and their dependents, veterans, narcotic addicts, Indians, and merchant seamen. State hospitals may specialize in care for the emotionally ill or the mentally retarded, or may be general hospitals such as those associated with a state-supported medical school. Most local city or county hospitals offer general medical care. Funds for these hospitals are provided by state and local taxes and/or federal taxes.

Voluntary Hospitals

Voluntary hospitals are private hospitals set up on a nonprofit basis. They provide inpatient beds for more than two-thirds of all hospital admissions in this country. Established by local communities, charitable organizations, churches, or philanthropic individuals, they are run by governing boards, usually selected from the community. They receive their funding from patients, insurance carriers such as Blue Cross, or government programs such as Medicare and Medicaid. New construction may be underwritten by local organizations or be funded in part by federal funds.

Proprietary Hospitals

Owned and administered by individuals or corporations, proprietary hospitals are set up to make a profit. Some are even established by real estate promoters and then leased to physicians at no construction cost to the community. Proprietary hospitals often have a questionable reputation. They tend to prefer the most profitable types of hospital cases, while taking few, if any, charity cases. The majority of these hospitals are small and only about one-third of them are accredited.

Accreditation of Hospitals

In 1952 a Joint Commission on Accreditation of Hospitals (JCAH) was set up to judge the operations of hospitals. It is sponsored by the American Hospital Association, the American Medical Association, the American College of Surgeons, and the American College of Physicians. It sets up national standards for hospital care, accredits hospitals meeting these standards, and periodically reviews accredited hospitals. To qualify, the hospital must have a tissue review committee that reviews the pathology of tissue removals and transfusions, and physician committees that review the surgical procedures and medical care of the hospital's physicians and take disciplinary action if required. Upon application, a hospital is thoroughly examined for cleanliness, laboratory operations, food handling, records, as well as the practice of its staff physicians. The hospital may be accredited for one or two years depending upon how well it qualifies.

It is increasingly important to have JCAH accreditation. A nonaccredited hospital may not train interns, residents, or nurses. Some medical insurance companies have refused to make payments to nonaccredited hospitals. Today, hospitals representing over 89 percent of the country's total hospital bed space are accredited. Most of these hospitals are voluntary ones.

Choosing a Hospital

If a person has the choice of selecting between two or more hospitals, how does he or she go about choosing? To get the best in health care, there are three questions that should be asked.

1. *Is the hospital accredited?* Accreditation by the JCAH does not guarantee a first-rate hospital, but it will mean that certain minimal standards have been met.

2. *Is it a teaching hospital?*   Hospitals which train medical and postgraduate students tend to provide better medical service; the higher the level of this teaching, the better the service. The best hospitals are those associated with medical schools. Here one should find medical specialists as instructors and qualified resident physicians training in the specialties.

3. *Who owns the hospital?*   Is it a voluntary (nonprofit) hospital or a proprietary (profit) one. A voluntary hospital is generally preferred since its operation rests in a community board of trustees rather than with the "owners" of a proprietary hospital, where quality will more directly relate to a desire for profit.

Decisions Before Entering a Hospital

Even though a hospital may provide qualified service, a patient must be satisfied that it is the best place to obtain the needed services. In some cases a nursing home might be better suited for providing care; especially for the elderly who often have strong aversions to entering a hospital. Cost is a consideration, even for those holding hospitalization insurance. Hospital care is more expensive than that from a nursing home. Medicare insurance, for example, provides for more days of paid care in a nursing home than in a hospital.

As to whether or not to enter a hospital, the recommendation of a physician can be relied upon. In fact, most hospitals will not admit a non-accident patient unless recommended by a physician.

Upon admission to a hospital the patient faces certain decisions. He or she may have a choice between a ward, semiprivate, or private room. Wards cost less per day, but also provide the patient with less privacy. Room selection should depend upon the nature of the illness, the patient's personal requirements, and ability to pay.

Summary

I. Modern Medicine

  A. Goals

    1. Available to *all* people

    2. Top priority given to *preventing* disease

    3. *Whole* person must be ministered to

    4. *Research* into unconquered diseases must be continued

  B. Problems faced by today's physician

    1. Current shortage of 50,000 physicians

      a. Only one physician for every 804 people

      b. More physicians in urban areas than rural

2. More specialists today and fewer family physicians

3. With less physician-patient contact and greatly refined techniques, there is great need for improved communication by physician with the patient

4. Greater hospital use by physicians has reduced their contact with home and knowledge of whole patient

C. Changes in medical practice

1. Concern over need to de-emphasize narrow specialties and re-emphasize general medicine

2. Need for further expansion of health insurance coverage, particularly among low-income families

3. Increasing numbers of physicians practicing together in medical groups or clinics in which certain services are shared

II. Choosing a Physician

A. Requirements to practice

1. Four years of college training, four years of medical school, one year of hospital internship

2. Licensed by a board of medical examiners after passing a state or national examination

3. Although not required, preferable for physician to belong to local and county medical societies

B. A family physician

1. Everyone should have a physician he or she can regard as a personal or family physician

2. General Practitioner (GP)

a. Only 16 percent of all physicians in the U.S. are general practitioners

b. In addition to regular medical school training and hospital internship, many have taken one or two additional years of training

c. The difficulty faced in keeping abreast with new medical information and techniques has led to the conception of the new medical specialty of Family Practice

3. Family Practice

a. Training consists of three or four years of graduate work in addition to regular medical training

b. Training may emphasize internal medicine, psychiatry, surgery, obstetrics, or pediatrics

c. To qualify as a specialist, board examination given by the American Academy of Family Practice must be passed

d. Main goal is to provide physicians who can take care of most of the patient-family illnesses and injuries

4. General internist

a. Must have completed six years of training after medical school and passed examination by American Board of Internal Medicine

b. Trained primarily in diagnosing

c. Among specialists, may serve as a family physician

C. The specialties

1. To be a recognized specialist, physician must be a *board diplomate* (pass the examinations) in chosen specialty

2. Internal medicine—internal diagnosis

3. Obstetrics and Gynecology—pregnancy, childbirth, and women's diseases

4. Pediatrics—infant and child care

5. Surgery—surgical corrections of physical conditions

6. Psychiatry—emotional disturbances

7. Pathology—the study of the disease process and identification of causes of particular maladies

D. Osteopathy

1. Field of medicine combining both use of medicine and physical manipulation

2. Osteopath qualified to serve as a family physician

E. Types of practice

1. Traditionally, physician practiced alone in own offices

2. Tendency now for them to form groups which may combine services such as lab facilities, nursing, and bookkeeping

F. Selecting the right physician

1. Consider reputation of physician

a. Contact local accredited hospital for names and addresses of physicians who practice there

b. Check their education credentials with a local or county medical society, local hospital, or in the *AMA Directory* or *Directory of Medical Specialists*

2. Visit office of physician and make appointment

a. Should be within easy commuting distance

b. Should be neat, clean, and orderly

      c. Discuss any patient-physician questions you have

      d. Choose a physician you feel comfortable with

G. Patient-physician relationship

  1. Patient entitled to receive careful, professional service

  2. Physician should keep patient well informed and pursue preventive medicine.

  3. Patient always entitled to seek further consultation with other physicians

  4. Patient should completely understand physician's fee schedule and discuss it with the physician in case of hardship

  5. Patient should follow instructions exactly and show confidence in the physician

H. Chiropractic

  1. Based on belief in impaired nerve function as basic cause of disease

  2. Treatment based on x-ray, physical manipulation, and diet

  3. Training usually four to six years beyond high school

  4. Chiropractor must not be considered a family physician

I. Dentistry

  1. Training consists of four years beyond college

  2. Majority of dentists are in general practice

  3. The number of dentists per population in the U.S. has decreased since 1950

J. Nursing

  1. Nursing team led by professional or registered nurse (R.N.)

  2. Training requires two to four years beyond high school

  3. Number of nurses in the U.S. in terms of the population is increasing

III. Facilities for patient care

A. Nursing Homes

  1. Provide health services for patients who are elderly, convalescent, or chronically ill

  2. In selecting, check accreditation, fee rates, proximity, availability of openings, and general reputation

B. Hospitals

  1. Provide complete medical facilities for various kinds of illnesses

  2. Centralized facilities enable physicians to see many patients in one place where the care is the best available

C. Kinds of hospitals

1. Governmental—set up for military personnel, dependents, Indians, merchant seamen, veterans, and certain illnesses by federal, state, or local governments

2. Voluntary—public non-profit hospitals which provide for more than two-thirds of all hospital admissions in the United States

3. Proprietary—owned and administered by individuals or corporations to make a profit

D. Accreditation of hospitals

1. Joint Commission on Accreditation of Hospitals accredits those hospitals meeting certain standards

2. Important for patients to select only accredited hospitals

E. Choosing a hospital

1. Is the hospital accredited

2. Is it a teaching hospital

3. Who owns the hospital

F. Decisions before entering a hospital

1. Patient must be satisfied it is best place to obtain needed treatment

2. Patient must choose type of room and whether or not he or she can meet its cost; nature of illness may dictate type of room

Questions for Review

1. List several of the goals of modern medicine.

2. What are some of the problems facing physicians in the 1970s?

3. Some people complain about the difficulty of obtaining the services of a physician. Give at least three reasons why a person living in a rural area might be justified in feeling this way.

4. Physicians have been able to treat greater numbers of patients through certain improvements in medical practice. In what ways have physicians been able to make better use of their time?

5. What training must a person complete before being entitled to be called an M.D. and practice medicine? In what ways might it be reassuring to a patient to know that the physician is a member of a local and county medical society?

6. In seeking family care, a person may consider either a GP or a specialist in family practice or internal medicine. Compare the three in terms of length of training, emphasis of training, and ways in which the training of each might restrict the physician's practice.

7. To what sort of specialist might one go for treatment or care of: emotional illness, pregnancy, disease unique to women, a broken arm, immunization for childhood diseases, eye diseases, rectal troubles, a nose ailment?

8. Some physicians incorrectly call themselves specialists. How can a person confirm that a given physician is indeed a certified specialist?

9. What is the history of osteopathy? Is it safe to consider osteopaths as family physicians? Why have some members of the medical profession raised questions regarding osteopathy?

10. If a person were to move into an unfamiliar community, what steps should be taken to locate a physician who will agree to provide medical care?

11. What steps should be taken to assure the strongest patient-physician relationship?

12. The title "doctor" is applied to both a physician and a chiropractor. For what reasons should a chiropractor not be considered as a family physician?

13. Distinguish between the services provided by hospitals, clinics, and nursing homes.

14. There are different sorts of hospitals. Compare governmental, voluntary, and proprietary hospitals in terms of ownership, control, kinds of care provided, size, and accreditation.

15. What does JCAH stand for? When was it started and by whom, and what was it set up to do? What must a hospital do to win recognition by JCAH?

16. A person should find answers to what three questions in making the best choice of a hospital?

Chapter 3

SELECTING HEALTH PRODUCTS

The proper selection of health-related products is more important than that of any other type of consumer goods. Not only can much money be wasted on ineffective products, but a person's health, or even his life, may depend upon his getting proper treatment for diseased conditions and avoiding the use of dangerous products. It is essential that self-treatment not be attempted when the services of a physician are needed.

Dangers of Self-Diagnosis and Self-Treatment

Attempts at self-diagnosis and self-treatment of all manner of health problems seem to be a great American tradition. There are several possible explanations for the tendency to "play doctor." As the country was being settled, doctors were very few and transportation was very poor, so self-treatment was a necessity. Even today, most physicians are very busy, appointments are difficult to get, and, for many people, the cost of proper medical care is discouraging. For many residents of rural areas and ethnic ghetto areas of large cities, transportation to medical facilities remains a problem. In addition to these factors, there is the continuing barrage of advertisements for self-treatment products for ailments of every description. Is it any surprise, then, that so many people still attempt self-treatment?

There are very real dangers in attempting self-diagnosis and self-treatment of any kind of symptom. The most serious risk is that a major (even life-threatening) disorder can easily be misdiagnosed as some common, minor problem and be treated as such. For example, a person who tried self-treatment might take cough drops when he actually had tuberculosis or lung cancer. Not only would the self-treatment be ineffective and possibly harmful, but proper medical treatment would be delayed, perhaps even until "too late."

Another danger in self-treatment is that not all home remedies and nonprescription drugstore products are completely safe to use. Some are dangerous when used in excessive amounts, in the presence of certain physical disorders, or in combination with other medicines.

When Is a Physician Needed?

It should be apparent by now that, in addition to the question of which products to select, there is always the question of whether any product should be selected without the consultation of a physician.

Obviously, people should not run to a physician for every little scrape, bruise, ache, or pain. If they did, our entire system of medical care would be swamped overnight and the doctors would be unable to take care of the more serious problems. How can we know, then, which of the hundreds of different symptoms that can develop require the services of a physician? There are several circumstances under which a physician should always be consulted:

1. *Severe symptoms.* Any type of attack in which the symptoms are severe or alarming should obviously receive prompt medical attention.

2. *Prolonged symptoms.* Any symptoms that persist day after day should be checked by a physician, even though the symptoms are minor. Serious chronic disorders are often revealed through persistent minor symptoms.

3. *Repeated symptoms.* Symptoms, even though minor, that recur time after time should be reported to a physician because, like prolonged symptoms, they may indicate a serious problem.

4. *Unusual symptoms.* Any symptoms which seem to be unusual, such as unusual bleeding, mental changes, weight gains or losses, digestive changes, or fatigue call for a visit to a physician.

5. *If in doubt.* If you are not sure whether you need to see a physician or not, the safest action is to see one. If there is a serious problem, it can be corrected in its early stages; if there is no problem, then you have paid a very small price for your peace of mind.

Health Products

Aspirin

Aspirin is probably the most effective medical substance which can be bought without a prescription today. Aspirin, often disguised under its chemical name of *acetylsalicylic acid,* is the principal active ingredient of literally hundreds of nonprescription remedies. In many of these preparations, aspirin is the *only* effective ingredient, but their cost may be many times that of plain aspirin tablets. When advertisements refer to the "pain reliever that doctors recommend most," they mean aspirin.

Aspirin has several beneficial properties. Its most common use is as a pain reliever, especially for headaches and muscular pains. It also has the ability to reduce fever and inflammation. For most people, aspirin may act as a mild sedative.

The "glorified aspirin" products often contain aspirin, phenacetin, and caffeine (APC compounds), aspirin and caffeine, or just aspirin with a buffering agent. These products have been shown to be no more effective for most persons than plain aspirin, though some people feel that buffers may reduce stomach irritation. Several products which originally contained phenacetin no longer contain this substance. Effective in the relieving of pain and reducing of fever, larger doses of phenacetin over a prolonged period can produce kidney damage.

Patients receiving large amounts of aspirin over long periods may develop a toxicity known as "salicylism," indicated by nausea, vomiting, ringing in the ears, hearing trouble, gastric bleeding, blood loss, vertigo, allergic reactions, and severe headache (which of course is not relieved by taking more aspirin). Although the moderate use of aspirin is generally safe, even here there are certain precautions to follow in its use. A few people suffer allergic reactions to aspirin (such as hives); other people find that aspirin causes stomach irritation. The stomach irritation (but not the allergy) can often be prevented by the presence of food in the stomach. The dosage recommended on the label should not be exceeded. Dosages above this level are not more effective and may be harmful.

Finally, aspirin should be used over long periods of time only on the recommendation of a physician, since it might otherwise be used to relieve the symptoms of a serious disorder which needs medical attention.

Aspirin is among the most common causes of poisoning of young children. It is important that aspirin, like any other medication, be kept where children cannot get to it, preferably in a locked cabinet. Specially flavored children's aspirin is a particular problem, since children will eat it as candy. Manufacturers are now required to use lids that prevent children from opening the bottles, but aspirin should still be carefully kept out of the reach of children. Some authorities even recommend splitting adult aspirin tablets for use with children rather than keeping the flavored aspirin in the house.

A compound that is similar in its actions to aspirin is acetaminophen. It is contained in more than 60 over-the-counter and prescription products, such as Excedrin and Tylenol. Appearing to have little toxicity, it is said to be safer for people with aspirin allergy or bleeding disturbances. When acetaminophen is combined with aspirin, as in Excedrin, these advantages, of course, are lost.

Remedies for Coughs and Colds

Every year new "miracle" cold remedies are offered to the public in massive advertising campaigns, only to drop quietly out of the market a few years later when their manufacturers release newer "miracles." The fact remains that despite the many advances in other fields of medicine, there is still no way to prevent or cure the common cold.

To put cough and cold remedies into their proper perspective, one needs to understand that a cold is caused by a *virus* and that, to date, only limited progress has been made toward producing drugs that will cure virus infections. In fact, no drug which will control the cold-producing viruses has yet been developed. A cough is a reflex action caused by the presence of foreign matter or other irritation within the respiratory system. The purpose of coughing is to remove the irritant. Cough and cold remedies may give symptomatic relief by deadening the cough reflex, opening a stuffed nose, or reducing fever, but they do not get at the base cause of the trouble.

By eliminating the symptoms, but not their source, the cough and cold remedies may, in the long run, prove harmful. For example, they tempt a person with a cold to go on with normal activities instead of going to bed for twenty-four hours. This rest period, early in the course of a cold, can often hasten recovery and prevent secondary infections and other complications. The result of "fighting" a cold is often secondary bacterial infection of the middle ear, sinus cavities, or lungs. Coughs can be the result of many serious conditions which need medical treatment rather than just a deadening of the cough reflex. For example, a cough could indicate tuberculosis, pneumonia, other infections of the lungs or bronchioles, or lung cancer.

The reputations of many products for "curing" colds come from the fact that most colds are gone in less than a week. If a cold lasts beyond a week, it is probably due to secondary bacterial infection and should be treated by a physician. Antibiotics have no effect upon the virus phase of a cold, but may be useful in clearing up the secondary infections. The cold sufferer should not pressure his doctor to prescribe antibiotics unless there is definite evidence of bacterial infection.

Most cold remedies contain an *analgesic* (aspirin, phenacetin, acetaminophen, or salicylamide) which can give relief from fever, aches, and pains. Many contain an *antihistamine* to dry up the mucous membranes in the nose and a *sympathomimetic*, or nasal decongestant (most effective if applied directly to the mucous membranes by means of a spray or nose drops (Table 3.1).

Antihistamines counteract the fluid release from cells that occurs during colds and allergy attacks. While this may relieve the effects of a cold and certain allergies; antihistamines do not cure the cold. If they seem to cure it, there is a possibility that the actual problem was an allergy and not a cold at all. Antihistamines very commonly produce side effects such as dizziness and drowsiness, so they should not be taken when driving a car or operating machinery.

Sympathomimetics affect the blood supply to the swollen linings of the nose and throat, but can cause major side effects on the cardiovascular system resulting in increased heart action, jitteriness, nervousness, and tachycardia (abnormally rapid heart beat). Diabetics should avoid them since they may raise blood sugar; patients with rapid or irregular heart action are advised against them; they may intensify high blood pressure and nervousness.

Products for the Mouth

We are concerned here with the multitude of products offered for the care of the teeth and the prevention of "bad breath." Few products have been advertised more heavily than certain toothpastes, mouthwashes, and other remedies for bad breath. This "hard sell" has led to an almost neurotic concern among many people for the state of their breath.

Bad Breath

Let us first consider the causes of bad breath. As with most other symptoms, there are many causes, only a few of which can be remedied by mouthwashes, toothpastes, and similar products. Breath odors may arise in the mouth, nose, throat, or lungs. Odors arising in the mouth are obviously more readily remedied than those arising in the lungs. Among the most common causes of breath odors are food particles which remain in the mouth and on the teeth for long periods of time and are broken down by putrefying bacteria. The same process, incidentally, is important in causing tooth decay.

The first step in preventing bad breath is to thoroughly clean the mouth after eating. This is especially important before going to bed at night. The best way to clean the mouth is, of course, to thoroughly brush the teeth and rinse the mouth well with plain water. Also useful in cleaning the mouth when brushing is impossible are dental floss, soft balsa-wood toothpicks, chewing gum (preferably sugarless), or just rinsing with plain water. Antiseptic mouthwashes are claimed to prevent mouth odors by killing the bacteria that decay stray food particles, but their antiseptic effect is rather short-term. While they do wash away food particles, so does plain water.

TABLE 3.1. Ingredients of Some Over-the-Counter Cough and Cold Preparations

	Analgesic					
	Aspirin	Acetamino-phen	Phen-acetin	Sali-cylam-ide	antihist-amine	sympatho-mimetic
Allerest Tabl.					X	X
Amphenol		X				
APC	X		X			
Bromo-Seltzer			X			
C-3						X
Contac					X	X
Cope					X	
Coricidin	X				X	X
Coricidin D	X				X	X
Dristan	X				X	X
Empirin Compound	X		X			
Excedrin	X			X		
Flavihist				X	X	X
4-Way Cold Tablets	X				X	X
Nyquil						X
Pertussin Plus					X	X
Robitussin A-C					X	
Romex					X	X
Sinarest					X	X
Sin-Off	X				X	X
Sinustat			X			X
Sinutab			X		X	X
Super-Anahist	X					X
Super-Anahist	X					X
Vicks Formula 44					X	X
Vicks Sinex					X	

The breath odors that come from eating onions and garlic and from smoking do not arise in the mouth but in the lungs. The odors of onions and garlic are absorbed into the blood from the intestines, carried by the blood to the lungs, and then excreted by the lungs into the breath. No kind of toothpaste, mouthwash, or other product can do more than just mask the offensive odor with a more pleasant odor such as mint or clove. Only time can eliminate the odor-causing substances from the blood; and only time, not mouthwash, can eliminate the odor-causing tobacco products from the lungs of smokers.

Other cases of bad breath are due to bacterial infections of the nose, throat, or teeth. Of course, a physician should be consulted for the treatment of such infections.

A bad taste in the mouth does not necessarily mean bad breath, nor does the absence of a bad taste prove that the breath is sweet. There is generally no way for an individual to know whether the breath is bad or not.

In summary, the best way to prevent bad breath is to keep the mouth clean, treat infections promptly, avoid onions and garlic, and avoid smoking.

Tooth Decay

Almost every brand of toothpaste is claimed to be the very best for the prevention of tooth decay. Are there really differences between them? Let us start by reviewing the causes of tooth decay. Basically, tooth decay comes from the destruction of the enamel on the surface of the tooth by acids. The acid which most violently attacks tooth enamel is *lactic acid*. Other acids may cause etchings on the enamel but lack the destructive action of lactic acid. Lactic acid is formed by the metabolic action of several kinds of tooth bacteria upon sugars from foods and drinks.

Dental research has shown that approximately 96 percent of all the harmful bacteria within the mouth live in the tiny crevice near the gum line between the tooth and gum. The damage done is not related to the *number* of bacteria present, but rather to their state of organization. It has been found that bacteria must be organized or clumped together in tiny colonies or clusters called *bacterial plaques* before they are capable of producing harmful effects such as decay, tender and bleeding gums, and foul breath. But the presence of bacteria alone in a disorganized or unclumped state produces no harmful effects. Once the bacteria have been disorganized, it takes twenty-four to thirty hours for them to reorganize.

The bacterial action suggests how a person might prevent tooth decay. If once each day a person disorganizes the bacteria in the mouth, he or she should be free from decay and gum problems such as pyorrhea. This should be done through a thorough brushing of the teeth and the use of dental floss. Since some people do not do a thorough brushing job, brushing after each meal improves the chances of disturbing all of the bacterial colonies. The use of a toothpaste or powder in brushing makes the task more pleasant but does little to improve the effectiveness of the brushing. Putting all advertising aside, the basic ingredients of toothpastes and powders are abrasives, detergents, and flavoring, and in several, stannous fluoride. Toothpastes do not kill the acid-forming bacteria, nor do they neutralize the decay-producing acids. Flossing should be done between each tooth and in the crevice around each tooth. Some people use disclosing wafers, little tablets of food coloring that color the plaque areas so a person can tell where plaque is heaviest, to check the effectiveness of their oral hygiene.

It has been well established that fluorides make tooth enamel more resistant to decay. Fluorides are available to the teeth in drinking water, by topical application to the surface of the effected area, as applied by a dentist or dental hygienist, or as applied in several toothpastes. The water supplies of some localities naturally contain adequate amounts of fluorides; many municipalities add it where the water supplies are deficient in it; it may be applied to the teeth in a dentist's office. Sodium fluoride, a form contained in drinking water, is especially effective with newly erupted teeth. Stannous fluoride, a form contained in several brands of toothpaste, is effective in causing some degree of hardening of the enamel in adults. In areas where the water supply contains adequate amounts of fluoride, the fluoride contained in a toothpaste is of little additional value. Excess amounts of fluoride, although not harmful, tend to cause a discoloration of the enamel.

To summarize the prevention of tooth decay: most harmful bacteria live in the crevice between the gum and the tooth; bacteria have to be organized to be harmful; and, once disorganized, it takes twenty-four to thirty hours for the bacteria to reorganize. Once each day floss the surface of each tooth, especially under the gum line; thoroughly brush the teeth, with particular attention to the tongue sides of the teeth and the cheek surfaces of the back teeth; and rinse the mouth vigorously afterwards to remove the bacteria which have been dislodged. Professional cleaning by a dentist or dental hygienist once or twice a year, depending upon one's particular mouth chemistry, is essential. This should be accomplished with full mouth x-rays every few years to examine for hard-to-see decay. This should guarantee that tooth loss does not become a problem later in life.

Remedies for the Digestive System

Indigestion

Considering the eating habits of the average person and the emotional stresses to which we are subjected, it is no surprise that a multitude of products are promoted for the treatment of "indigestion." Actually, indigestion has no precise meaning. The word is applied to a variety of symptoms, including nausea, pain in the chest or abdomen, gas, and belching. These symptoms can result from any one of many minor or serious problems.

Among the minor causes of indigestion are overeating, drinking too much, highly spiced or greasy foods, and emotional upsets. In such cases, when the cause is definitely known and the attacks are infrequent, it is generally safe to use any of the common brands of indigestion remedies. The main action of these pills and powders is to neutralize the excess stomach acid that builds up when undigested food lies in the stomach.

But indigestion may also be a symptom of a serious hidden illness. If indigestion is frequent, painful, or has no obvious cause, then a physician should be consulted. Such types of indigestion could indicate ulcers, cancer, internal infections, or one of many other serious disorders.

Constipation

For many years, Americans seemed to be obsessed with the supposed need for a daily bowel movement (defecation). If a day's bowel movement was missed, drastic measures were often taken to "restore regularity." This concern was reinforced by laxative advertisements which predicted very grave results from "irregularity." It is to be hoped that this interest in the frequency of one's bowel movements is dying out as it becomes more widely known that a daily bowel movement is *not necessary*.

If the sales of laxatives go down, however, manufacturers are likely to respond with bigger and better advertising campaigns, so it is important to understand why laxatives should ordinarily *not* be used. In the first place, there are millions of people in perfect health who defecate only once every two or three days, or even less often, with absolutely no harmful effects. The most common complication of infrequent defecation is that too much water may be absorbed from the feces, leaving them hard and difficult or painful to pass (constipation).

There are several common causes of constipation. One of the most common causes is ignoring the urge to defecate. If defecation is postponed, the sensation of a full rectum passes. After the urge returns and leaves several times, the rectum may temporarily lose its sensitivity, so the feces are retained for long periods of time and too much water is absorbed. Then, when defecation is attempted, it is difficult.

Constipation can sometimes be caused by a diet that is too low in fruits and vegetables. Most fruits and vegetables contain a certain amount of indigestible material (called roughage) which stimulates the muscles of the rectum. Some fruits also contain specific chemicals that act as laxatives.

Among users of laxatives, the laxatives themselves are very commonly the cause of constipation. This may come about in several ways. First, a powerful laxative may empty the intestine so thoroughly that several days may go by before enough feces accumulate to cause a need for defecation. But by then the person may have become concerned and taken more laxative. Thus, a normal bowel movement may never occur. The use of laxatives irritates the wall of the rectum so that in time its muscular reflexes are reduced to the point that constipation becomes chronic.

No specific treatments for constipation should be used unless they have been prescribed by a physician. This applies to all types of laxatives, as well as enemas and suppositories. If hard feces make defecation painful, the condition can often be remedied by including more fruits and vegetables in the diet, drinking more water, and getting more exercise. If the problem still persists, a physician should be consulted.

Hemorrhoids (Piles)

Hemorrhoids are varicose (swollen) veins in the rectum or around the anus. Hemorrhoids within the rectum are called internal; those around the anus are called external. Perhaps two out of three adults have some degree of piles. If piles are severe enough to cause discomfort, a physician should be consulted. The various highly advertised remedies are of doubtful value and their use is often the cause of further complications, such as intense itching.

Products for the Eyes

Eye Washes

Many physicians warn against the self-treatment of the eyes with any kind of commercial eye wash or eye drops. The natural flow of tears through the eye is the best means of cleaning the eye of dust, dirt, and other irritating material. Like many kinds of self-treatment remedies, eye washes may be used to try to relieve the symptoms of serious eye disorders which really need prompt treatment by a physician. If any of the symptoms for which eye washes are advertised (red eyes, sore eyes) last for more than a day or two, the eyes should be immediately examined by a physician.

Eyeglasses

Eyeglasses should not be purchased from variety stores or by mail order. Anyone having difficulty with his or her vision should have a thorough eye examination by an eye specialist. The problem may need treatment other than glasses, and in any event, glasses should be carefully fitted to the specific eyes of the individual and not just purchased at random.

To reduce the hazard of eye injury from shattering eyeglass lenses, the FDA now requires that eyeglass and sunglass lenses be resistant to breaking upon impact, as determined by a standardized physical test (the dropping, from a measured distance, of a metal ball onto the glass being tested; glass withstanding the impact is judged safe by FDA standards). Contact lenses are not covered by these regulations, nor are the various forms of goggles and face masks such as those used in skiing and swimming.

Contact Lenses

Contact lenses are small plastic lenses that ride on a thin layer of tears directly over the cornea and under the eyelids (Fig. 3.1). Recent improvements in their construction have increased their popularity. Practically invisible when worn, contact lenses are widely used by people in sports and entertainment and by many others who dislike the appearance of regular glasses.

Contact lenses cannot be used by everyone. Certain types of visual defects can be corrected satisfactorily with "contacts"; others cannot. Contact lenses must be placed in the eye and taken out daily. They are easily lost, and some people find them too irritating to wear at all. Recently, soft contact lenses have become available. They are made of a soft plastic material that is absorptive to water and maintains a 36 percent water content when being worn. Somewhat more comfortable, they are particularly useful for persons whose eyes are supersensitive to the hard contact lenses.

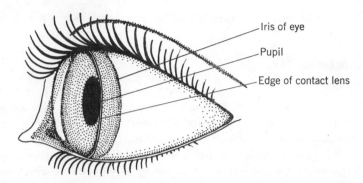

Figure 3.1 *Contact lens, floating on a layer of tears over the cornea of the eye.*

Contact lenses must be properly fitted to the eye by a qualified optometrist or ophthalmologist. It may take many adjustments before they can be worn comfortably. This makes contact lenses expensive. There are those who advertise contact lenses at lower prices, but these individuals or organizations are often unwilling to make the necessary adjustments to make the lenses fit properly. Poorly fitted contact lenses are very uncomfortable and may even damage the cornea.

Sunglasses

Bright sunlight or glare can cause squinting, eyestrain, and headache, and may contain harmful amounts of ultraviolet rays which can gradually damage the lens and retina of the eyes. Sunglasses can reduce the discomfort of bright sun and screen out much of the ultraviolet light. Another reason for wearing sunglasses is that vision during the early evening hours is considerably reduced if the eyes have been exposed to bright sunlight during the day. This is hazardous if one is driving.

The prices of sunglasses range from very inexpensive to very expensive. It is wise to pay a little more and get a good pair of sunglasses. There are several requirements for a good pair of sunglasses. First, they should be fairly dark. Second, they should be properly ground, as optical flaws will create eyestrain and headache just as severe as that produced by the bright sun. Figure 3.2 illustrates a simple way of determining the optical quality of a pair of sunglasses before buying them. A person who normally wears prescription lenses should have sunglasses ground to his prescription or get the type that clip over his glasses.

Sunglasses should *never* be worn for night driving or for looking directly at the sun.

Pills for Sleeping, Waking, and Relaxing

Since most drugs that really affect the mind are under strict government control and are legally available by prescription only, you may have wondered just what is in the nonprescription pills so openly advertised as being useful for sleeping or relaxing, relieving nervous tension, and staying awake.

Pills for Sleeping or Relaxing

Nonprescription pills for sleeping or relieving nervous tension are entirely different from the pills a doctor might prescribe for the same conditions.

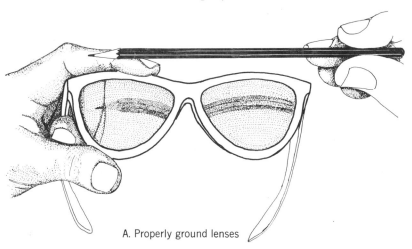

A. Properly ground lenses

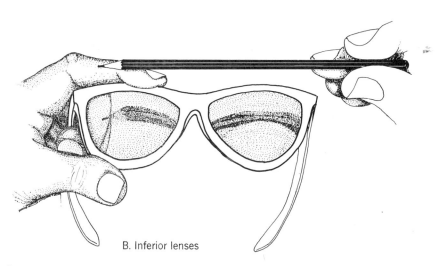

B. Inferior lenses

Figure 3.2 *Simple test for optical quality of sunglasses. (A) properly ground lenses reflect without distortion. (B) poorly ground lenses reflect distorted image and transmit distorted image to the eye.*

These advertised pills generally take advantage of one of the side effects of the antihistamine drugs. Antihistamines, which can be sold without a prescription, are useful in relieving the symptoms of certain types of allergies and are commonly contained in remedies for colds.

Certain of the antihistamines have the side effects of producing drowsiness, which may be rather severe in some people. For this reason, these antihistamines are sold as nonprescription sleeping pills. For many persons, these sleeping pills will really produce drowsiness; for some people, they may be a psychological aid to sleep (since most sleeplessness is psychological); and for some, there will be no effect at all. For a few other people, the antihistamines act as stimulants, producing nervousness and sleeplessness, thus contributing to the problem for which they were taken. The nonprescription sleeping and relaxing pills often contain small amounts of other mild sedatives, but not enough to have any real effect.

If nonprescription sleeping pills are tried, they should be taken *exactly as directed on the label*. Higher dosages (perhaps even the recommended dosage) can produce various side effects such as a dry mouth, dizziness, blurred vision, incoordination, loss of appetite, and nervousness. You should never drive a car or operate machinery after taking any antihistamine drug.

Pills for Staying Awake

The pills that are advertised as helping you stay awake are usually based on caffeine. Caffeine, of course, is contained in coffee, tea, and cola drinks. Though not everyone reacts in the same way, many people do find that caffeine acts as a stimulant which can prevent sleep; caffeine also makes some people feel nervous ("coffee nerves"); so the sleep preventing pills will do for a person just what coffee does for them. The effect of one tablet is usually about equal to one cup of strong coffee.

The situations which justify taking these pills are rather limited. They do not serve as a substitute for sleep but merely relieve the symptom of sleepiness. Their use has been compared to "whipping tired horses." They may help you study for an extra hour or two, but beyond that your ability to learn drops considerably. They should not be used to extend night driving for more than an hour or two because driving becomes very dangerous beyond that point. A person who badly needs sleep may have dangerous hallucinations while driving or may just suddenly fall asleep at the wheel.

Cosmetics

The first 30 to 50 pages of *Seventeen,* or any other young person's magazine, leads through a tantalizing parade of cosmetic ads featuring beautiful people and equally appealing cosmetic products. The ads advise you on eliminating split, chipped nails; they introduce you to sexy-young smells, to waterproof eye shadow, to conditioners for long hair and to lip glossers. They tell of sweet earth fragrances that "nature wears herself," foams and lotions that give tans in three to five hours with or without sun, shampoos that replace the natural protein "stripped away" by coloring agents, sun damage, and harsh shampoos. Cosmetic ads may make exaggerated claims since, unlike drug ads, they do not have to show that their products are effective.

What's with this multimillion dollar industry? What exactly is a cosmetic? According to the federal Food, Drug, and Cosmetic Act, cosmetics are defined as "(1) articles intended to be rubbed, poured, sprinkled, or sprayed on, introduced into, or otherwise applied to the human body or any part thereof for cleansing, beautifying, promoting attractiveness, or altering the appearance, and (2) articles intended for use as a component of any such articles, except soaps." Today more than 80 products are considered to be cosmetics by the Food and Drug Administration.

Cosmetics may also be considered as drugs when they make claims to alter a body function. For example, a deodorant is regulated as a cosmetic, because it is intended only to prevent odor; but an antiperspirant is regulated as a drug because it is intended to actually reduce perspiration, which is a normal body function. If a cosmetic is looked upon as a drug, its ingredients must be listed as "active ingredients" and listed ahead of all other ingredients. This type of listing is found, for instance, on the labels of dandruff shampoos, hormone creams, antiperspirants, sunscreen products, and all medicated cosmetics.

Skin Conditioners

Since our skin and hair have such a great effect on our appearance, they deserve the best of care. Knowing that most people care about their appearance, manufacturers advertise a multitude of products with claims of handsomeness, beauty, and sex appeal. Some of these products are very good, some are just so-so, and some are actually harmful.

Skin is nourished by the blood and the way to make sure the necessary nutrients are available to the skin is to eat properly. Nutritional requirements for the skin are the same as for the rest of the body—a balanced diet of fruits, vegetables, meats, milk, and eggs provide the nutrients needed for healthy skin. Dry skin will benefit from a simple oil, cream, or lotion. Since hormones can be absorbed through the skin in quantities large enough to have side effects, hormone skin creams should be used only on the recommendation of a physician. Exotic ingredients such as orchid pollen, royal jelly, and turtle oil are of no special or cosmetic value.

Persons bothered by skin irritations may reduce or eliminate the irritation through some common sense practices. Underarm irritation may come from rubbing too hard when drying, as well as from a cosmetic/drug being used. Shaving too closely damages the skin. Clothing worn too tightly can chafe. Stiff, new clothing can also be a cause of skin irritation—especially some of the permanent-press clothes. When a product containing alcohol, which most deodorants contain, is applied to already irritated skin, a temporary burning sensation occurs.

A bothersome problem with both skin conditioners and eye cosmetics has been the presence of microorganisms, particularly the *Pseudomonas*. These are bacteria which, once in the body, may infect organs such as the kidneys and which are notably resistant to the effect of antibiotics. Because of these and other bacterial organisms, it is necessary to include preservatives in cosmetics, such as formaldehyde, mercuric compounds, and hexachlorophene. Minute amounts of formaldehyde have been found to cause skin sensitization. Hexachlorophene use was severely restricted in cosmetics and drugs after it was shown that it could be absorbed through the unbroken skin and could affect the nervous system.

Eye Cosmetics

Small amounts of carefully applied cosmetics can highlight a woman's appearance and emphasize certain features, but the heavy application of cosmetics does not improve the appearance and may damage the complexion.

Cosmetics should be used around the eyes with extreme care. Some women have had eyelashes fall out through careless use of eye cosmetics. Some cosmetics cause rashes or other skin reactions in some people (it is wise to test a new cosmetic on your arm or body before putting it on your face.).

More serious are possible eye infections brought on by the use and misuse of eye cosmetics. Preservatives are placed in eye products to retard the growth of hazardous bacteria. But during months of storage on the shelf of a pharmacy the preservatives may lose their ability to protect. Once the eye product is opened, microorganisms gain ready access to the cosmetic. Many women infect their eyes daily with eye cosmetics because of the high concentration of microorganisms growing in the products after they are opened and used.

The human eye is bathed with secretions which keep in balance the normal skin microorganisms migrating into the eye mucosa (underside of eyelid) and onto the eyeball surface. However, the introduction of large numbers of these same microorganisms which have grown in a contaminated eye product severely challenges these protective secretions. FDA studies have shown that if the cornea is scratched with a mascara brush or irritated by wearing contact lenses or using an eye-irritating shampoo, bacteria such as *Pseudomonas* (a type that can cause eye infections) infect the eye and pose a serious hazard to a person's vision. A scratch on the cornea (outer surface of the eyeball) allows the bacteria to invade and infect the cornea. Although some infections have caused blindness, most eye infections do not.

The problem remains, no matter how well the preservative works in an eye cosmetic, that if the product is misused by the consumer, infections can still develop. The FDA suggests the following precautions in the use of eye cosmetics:

1. Discontinue immediately the use of any eye product that causes irritation. If irritation persists, see a physician.

2. Recognize that your hands contain microorganisms that, if placed in the eye, could cause infections. Wash your hands before applying cosmetics to your eyes.

3. Make sure that any instrument you place in the eye area is clean.

4. Do not allow eye cosmetics to become covered with dust or contaminated with dirt or soil. Wipe off the container with a damp cloth if visible dust or dirt is present.

5. Do not use old containers of eye cosmetics. If you haven't used the product for several months, it's better to discard it and purchase a new one.

6. Do not spit into eye cosmetics. The microorganisms in your mouth may grow in the cosmetic and subsequent application to the eye may cause infection. Boiled water can be added to products which have thickened.

7. Do not share your cosmetics. Another person's microflora in your cosmetic can be hazardous.

8. Do not store cosmetics at temperatures above 85° F. Cosmetics held for long periods in hot cars, for example, are more susceptible to deterioration of the preservative.

9. Avoid using eye cosmetics if you have an eye infection or the skin around the eye is inflamed. Wait until the area is healed.

10. Take particular care in using eye cosmetics if you have any allergies.

11. When removing eye cosmetics, be careful not to scratch the eyeball or some other sensitive area.

These simple precautions should eliminate the causes of most eye infections introduced by cosmetics. They apply to the use of eye products for healthy eyes. Products used to correct deficiencies or injuries of the eye are considered drugs, and as such, must meet more rigorous standards. Eye drugs obtained by prescription are approved by the FDA for safety and effectiveness, including effective preservatives. By contrast, eye drugs sold over-the-counter without a prescription have not been precleared by the FDA for the presence of effective preservatives; they therefore require more caution on the part of the consumer.

Deodorants and Antiperspirants

The socially aware person wants his or her skin not only to look good, but to smell good, too. The body is equipped with two types of sweat glands— one responsible for much of the moisture of sweat (eccrine glands), the other for the odor (apocrine glands).

About three million tiny eccrine glands prevent the body from over- heating. They secrete a clear, odorless liquid of 99 percent water and one percent sodium chloride. When the water evaporates from the skin, it takes heat from the body but also keeps the skin moist and supple. The eccrine gland responds to two kinds of stimuli—thermal (heat) and emo- tional (fear, pain, tension, sexual excitement, etc.). Eccrine glands on the palms, soles, and underarms respond to both stimuli. Those on the rest of the body respond only to thermal stimulation, except in extreme emotional stimulation, which brings on a "cold sweat" over the whole body. Wetness alone does *not* cause body odor.

Apocrine glands serve no known useful purpose. Far fewer in num- ber than eccrine glands, they function primarily in hairy underarm regions. Present at birth, they begin to function when a person reaches puberty and respond only to emotional stimulation. Their activity reaches a peak with sexual maturity and diminishes with old age. When stimulated, they secrete a viscous, milky liquid composed of complex organic materials, which is decomposed by bacteria on the skin to form the smelly end- products known as "body odor" or "underarm odor." Such bacteria are normal on the skin and thrive in the warm, moist underarms.

Since sweating causes two problems—wetness and odor—two types of products are needed. The *deodorant* works against body odor; the *anti- perspirant* works against both wetness and body odor.

There are several ways to control body odor. You can wash organic material away before the bacteria can decompose it; you can try to mask the odor with a more pleasant odor (perfumes are used for this, but they are volatile and do not last); you can inhibit the growth of the bacteria by removing the moisture necessary for their growth (except that no products completely stop eccrine sweating); or you can kill the bacteria or inhibit their growth with antibacterial agents. Such agents stick to the skin even after washing; thus, deodorant effectiveness builds up over a period of days (or tapers off if use is discontinued). Antibacterial agents include zinc phenosulfonate and methylbenzethonium chloride.

The best way to control body odor is with a combination of methods. Regular use of a scented deodorant or antibacterial soap will keep you free from offensive body odor for at least 24 hours. Deodorants only kill or inhibit the bacteria; thus, a deodorant is not a substitute for washing.

Antiperspirants reduce the flow of perspiration from the eccrine gland through the use of metal salts such as aluminum or zirconium. They also reduce body odor through the use of antibacterial ingredients. The most common antiperspirant ingredients are aluminum chlorhydroxide (or chlorhydrate or hydroxychloride) and aluminum chloride. To be effective, an antiperspirant ingredient must penetrate the sweat duct. For the greatest antiperspirant action, apply the product when you are not already sweating. Instead of applying it immediately after a bath, when the body is warm, apply it when you are at rest and cool. Then lie down for a few minutes—you sweat least then and consequently the antiperspirant penetrates better.

Deodorants and antiperspirant deodorants are available in many forms—liquid, pads, creams, roll-ons, sticks, powders, and aerosols. Read the label to be sure the product is actually an antiperspirant. An antiperspirant must list its active ingredients; deodorants will be listing active ingredients beginning in 1976. If *active* ingredients are listed, the product is an antiperspirant (since it is looked upon as a drug by the FDA).

There are many misconceptions surrounding the problem of how to control sweating. For example, you do not need a deodorant more in summer than in winter, since apocrine (odor) sweating is about the same all year round. Stopping perspiration is not unhealthy—sweating is a method of regulating body temperature, not disposing of body wastes. You cannot become immune to one deodorant or antiperspirant product and need to change to another product—deodorants and antiperspirants do not lose effectiveness and people do not build up immunity to them. A perspiring person does not automatically have body odor—eccrine sweat is odorless. Men do not need a stronger deodorant than do women—the amount of apocrine secretion is about the same for both sexes (although unshaved hair under the arm tends to act as a collecting ground for decomposing body products and bacteria).

Other Deodorants

Foot deodorants help dry moisture, reduce perspiration, and give a soothing feeling. Although there are no apocrine glands on the foot, feet may smell when bacteria thrive in warm moist areas where dead skin cells are constantly being rubbed off and decomposed.

Two types of products are intended to reduce the problem of vaginal odor during menstruation. One type is intended for use directly on sanitary napkins; the other, for use on the external genital area. Both kill bacteria or inhibit their growth. Feminine hygiene sprays for use throughout the month are available. For those who use them here's a word of caution. Not only do they tend to irritate the vaginal area, they also are essentially unnecessary. They do little other than provide, for some women, a psychological reassurance that there is no noticeable vaginal odor, especially during the menstrual period.

Body deodorants reduce bacteria on the skin and leave a pleasant odor. Some come as dusting or aerosol powders to which an antibacterial agent has been added.

Products for Acne

Acne can be one of the most troublesome problems of youth. The skin appears greasy and it is marked by blackheads, red spots, and pus-filled pimples. The person with acne may feel self-conscious about it, though it probably looks worse to him than it does to other people. But severe cases of acne can leave scars that may last for years.

Many products are advertised for the treatment of acne, but none of these products are answers to the problem. Many cases of acne *can* be cleared with proper home care. There are several simple steps to this care.

1. *Proper diet is important.* The best diet for those fighting acne includes plenty of fruits, vegetables, and lean meats. To be avoided are sweet, starchy, and fatty foods.

2. *Cleanliness.* The heart of the acne problem is the overproduction of oil by the oil glands of the face, neck, back, and chest. The openings of these glands get clogged with oil and dirt, enlarge, and become infected with bacteria. Therefore, the face and other affected parts should be thoroughly washed three or four times a day with plenty of hot water and soap. A deodorant or disinfectant type of soap is valuable for inhibiting the infecting bacteria, as long as it does not irritate the skin. Gently rub the lather into the skin for several minutes to remove the excess oil. Rinse first with hot water to open the pores, then rinse again with cold water to close the pores. Over a period of time this will remove the blackheads and other types of plugged pores.

Girls should *not* try to clean their faces with creams in place of soap and water. This is the worst possible treatment for acne, since oil needs to be removed, not added. Cosmetics of all kinds should be used very sparingly, if at all. Many kinds of cosmetics contain fine particles which may clog the pores.

3. *Do not squeeze pimples or blackheads.* This often spreads the infection, enlarges the pimples, and may even force the bacteria into the blood. A pimple that has been squeezed or picked may leave a permanent scar.

If acne does not clear up with two or three weeks of the home care just described, then *consult a physician promptly.* If effective treatment is delayed too long, there may be some permanent scarring of the skin. While there are techniques for removing much of the scar tissue today, it is far better to prevent the scarring in the first place.

Suntans and Sunburns

Many lightly pigmented people feel that they look better with a suntan. Almost everyone experiences a feeling of well-being when warmed by the sun; yet the beneficial effects of the sun are almost nil, and there are in fact adverse effects.

If a person insists on getting a tan, there are several safety measures that can be taken. Human skins vary greatly in the amount of sun they can tolerate. Dark-skinned individuals have more immunity to sunburn than the fair-skinned; yet even the person who tans well must be careful to avoid sunburn at the beginning of the summer. The key is to start with short periods of exposure and work up to longer periods. For a person with light skin, the first exposure early in the season should not exceed 15 to 20 minutes for each side, front, and back. If you begin tanning later in the season, the length of first exposure should be even shorter. You can increase the exposure by about one-third each day. After a few days, exposures of several hours may be possible. Rays are reflected from sand and water, which means that you can burn even while sitting under an umbrella. You can burn on a hazy day as well.

Suntan preparations are of varying value. Many lotions contain chemicals called sunscreens that absorb (screen out) ultraviolet rays to some degree. The better lotions allow you to stay in the sun longer. They do not shut out all the radiation; if they did, you would never tan. Despite the claims of advertisements, there is no way to screen out the "burning rays" of the sun while admitting the "tanning rays," since they are one and the same. Read the label before purchasing any preparation. Paraminobenzoic acid, the salicylates, and benzophenone compounds are among the most effective sunscreens. Suntan lotions must be reapplied at least every two hours or after each swim. A word of caution—commercial sunburn preparations contain ingredients that may cause allergic skin reactions.

Those who like to tan very deeply every year should be aware of several possible effects of extreme long-term sun exposure. One is the development of premature wrinkles caused by the aging effects of ultraviolet rays on the skin. The skin may actually be made to look many years older than its true age. Another possible result is the development of skin cancer. Skin cancer is most common on the constantly exposed parts of the skin, such as the face, neck, and ears. It is more common among people who suntan with difficulty than among those who tan easily.

Skin care following sunbathing is important to prevent excessive drying. Apply an emollient lotion or cream to the skin after bathing or before retiring. If you get a sunburn, apply a soothing lotion or ointment, such as cold cream or baby oil, or a wet compress to relieve the pain. If the pain is excessive, or if extensive blistering is present, see a physician.

A word is in order on sunlamps. Sunlamps are widely used in the United States to improve the appearance of the skin. Some bathers want a ruddy outdoor appearance even in midwinter. Some feel that the contrast of a flashing white smile with a deep tan is extremely flattering.

Sunlamp bathers must be aware that ultraviolet radiation that tans and beautifies the skin can also cause painful sunburns and permanent eye damage. The biggest problem in using sunlamps is overexposure. Under some lamps one minute of ultraviolet radiation can be equivalent to one hour under the sun. Some purchasers of lamps do not read instructions; others read but fail to follow.

Here are some suggestions from the FDA for safe use of ultraviolet ray bulbs and sunlamps:

1. Upon purchase, read and observe all instructions carefully. If instructions are not permanently attached to the lamp, tape them to the lamp's base or stand so that they will not be lost and will be available to successive users.

2. Be precise in measuring exposure time and distance from the lamp. Use a tape measure, and use a timer with an alarm bell so that if attention wanders, you will be alerted immediately to over-exposure. Better still, purchase a sunlamp with a timing device to automatically turn off the lamp at a proper time.

3. Wear close-fitting eye protection.

4. Never stare directly at the lighted bulb.

5. Guard against mirrors that can reflect ultraviolet rays not only to the person using a sunlamp but also to persons nearby.

6. Never become so comfortable under a lamp that there is danger of becoming drowsy or falling asleep.

7. Remember that reading or similar activities under a sunlamp can be harmful to eyes.

8. Children should be carefully supervised under any form of ultra-violet light by responsible adults to guard against overexposure and insure that eye protection is worn.

Shampoos

The hair and scalp need to be washed frequently. The oil glands of the scalp are very active in most persons. The oil that these glands produce accumulates on the scalp and hair, becomes rancid and bad-smelling, causes the hair to look stringy, and contributes to acne as well.

The exact frequency with which hair should be washed depends on the amount of oil produced and the exposure to dirt. Many hair experts suggest weekly washing as a minimum, with twice-weekly washing recommended for those with a more oily scalp. A regular shampoo should be used. Bar soap may be difficult to rinse from the hair and the various dry and "instant" shampoos do not adequately clean the hair and scalp. Shampoos vary in their ability to remove oil. The person with an oily scalp needs a shampoo which removes much oil; while the person with a dry scalp should select a shampoo intended especially for that condition.

Dandruff

There is no single cause or sure cure for dandruff. Since the scalp normally loses dead cells from its surface, as does the rest of the skin, it is reasonable to expect at least some flaking of epidermis from the scalp. This is a perfectly normal and unavoidable condition. Excess dandruff, however, can be a real problem, usually falling into one of three basic types. The first of these is associated with a very dry scalp. It can often be helped by using a dry-scalp shampoo or hair-oil preparation. The second type results from too much oil, causing the dead skin cells to cling together in clusters, forming dandruff flakes. This type of dandruff may be helped by frequent shampooing. A third type of dandruff includes a thick oily crust or scales over the scalp. This may indicate an infection, so it should be checked by a physician.

The special dandruff-removing shampoos, which generally are more expensive than the regular products, seem to be little better than the plain shampoos for many people. While the special shampoos do apparently help in some cases, the treatment of dandruff remains a matter of trial and error.

Hair-Removal Products

Of the many methods of removing excess hair, the safest and simplest method is still by shaving with a safety razor or electric razor. This is the method normally used by men for shaving the beard and by most women for removing hair from the legs and underarms.

The various chemical hair-removal products require more care in their use. Any chemical that is strong enough to dissolve hair can also cause injury to the skin. If these products are allowed to remain on the skin too long, a severe chemical burn may result. These products can be quite damaging to the eyes, so they should never be used on the face, even though they may be advertised for that purpose.

Women sometimes wish to permanently remove excess facial hair. The only method of permanently removing hair is electrolysis. With this technique, a fine needle is inserted into the root of each hair (one by one) and an electric current is run down the needle until the hair root is destroyed. This method is safe and leaves no scars if the operator is adequately skilled. In order to select such a skilled operator, a recommendation should be obtained from a physician. Electrolysis is expensive.

Safe Use of Cosmetics

According to the FDA, today's cosmetics are among the safest products available to consumers; yet no rules and regulations or precautions by government or industry can protect the person who doesn't follow the label directions and warnings.

Following are some basic unwritten rules of good judgment that could keep a customer's experience with cosmetics off the "adverse reaction" list:

1. Read and follow all directions and warnings on the product. If patch testing (trying a portion of the product first on a very small area of your skin) is suggested for any product, don't neglect this measure to determine your sensitivity to the product. Furthermore, sensitivity can change: hair color, skin cream, or another type of product that should be patch tested may irritate you the next time you use it, even though it hasn't in the past. Your body chemistry is always changing.

2. Basic cleanliness—in other words, washing your hands before applying a cosmetic—is important not only to your skin and appearance, but also for maintaining a clean product. Another point to remember is to close containers after each use; dust and germs can easily settle into any product left uncovered.

3. Never borrow another person's cosmetics. You may be swapping trouble. Bacteria may have contaminated the other person's cosmetics.

4. When water must be added to a cosmetic before it can be used— such as cake eyeliner—it is a dangerous practice to substitute saliva for water. This can result in the transfer of bacteria from the mouth to the eye, causing an eye infection.

5. If you develop an adverse reaction, don't try to "wait it out." See your physician immediately. To speed diagnosis, take with you the cosmetic you suspect is causing your problem.

These actions are the consumer's own "voluntary program" for safety; they can be enforced only by the consumer at home.

Selecting Safe Toys

Although this chapter is entitled *Selecting Health Products,* it is proper that we give a few pointers for safe toy buying. Each year an estimated 700,000 injuries are caused by toys. The FDA has removed from sale over 800 types of toys, but the FDA can go only so far in protecting children from unsafe toys. Care in buying and parental supervision can reduce most toy injuries.

When choosing a toy for young children, make sure it:

1. Is too large to be swallowed.
2. Does not have detachable parts that can lodge in the windpipe, ears, or nostrils.
3. Is not apt to break easily into small pieces or leave jagged edges.
4. Does not have sharp edges or points.
5. Has not been put together with easily exposed straight pins, sharp wires, nails, etc.
6. Is not made of glass or brittle plastic

7. Is labeled "nontoxic"—avoid painted toys for infants who put playthings in the mouth.

8. Does not have parts which can pinch fingers or toes or catch hair.

Summary

I. Dangers of Self-diagnosis and Self-treatment

   A. Major problem may be misdiagnosed as minor disorder

   B. Proper medical treatment may be delayed

   C. Home remedies or nonprescription drugs may be dangerous in many circumstances

II. When Is a Physician Needed?

   A. Severe symptoms

   B. Prolonged symptoms

   C. Repeated symptoms

   D. Unusual symptoms

   E. If in doubt

III. Health Products

   A. Aspirin

      1. Is acetylsalicylic acid

      2. Is probably the most effective nonprescription drug

      3. Will relieve pain, reduce fever and inflammation, and may act as mild sedative for some people

      4. Recommended dosages should not be exceeded

      5. Must be kept out of reach of children

   B. Remedies for coughs and colds

      1. There is still no way to prevent or cure the common cold

      2. Many cold remedies are based on antihistamines which may cause dizziness or drowsiness, making driving dangerous if taken

   C. Tooth Decay

      1. Due to destruction of enamel by lactic acid formed by tooth bacteria

      2. Bacteria do their damage when organized in bacterial plaques

      3. Once bacteria have been disorganized by brushing, it takes 24–30 hours to reorganize

      4. Teeth should be thoroughly brushed at least once each day

5. Fluorides are especially effective in hardening enamel of newly erupted teeth, and somewhat effective on enamel of adult teeth

6. Every person should have teeth cleaned once or twice a year by a dentist or dental hygienist

D. Remedies for the digestive system

1. Indigestion—if frequent, painful, or has no obvious cause, a physician should be consulted

2. Constipation—no specific treatments should be used unless they have been prescribed by a physician

3. Hemorrhoids—if severe enough to cause discomfort, a physican should be consulted

E. Products for the eyes

1. Eyewashes—many physicians warn against any self-treatment of the eyes

2. Eyeglasses—should not be purchased from variety stores or by mail order

3. Contact lenses—must be properly fitted by a qualified optometrist or ophthalmologist

4. Sunglasses

    a. Should be worn in bright sunlight or glare

    b. Should be of good quality

    c. Should never be worn for night driving or for looking at the sun

F. Pills for sleeping, waking, and relaxing

1. Pills for sleeping or relaxing

    a. Generally contain antihistamines

    b. Must be taken exactly as directed on the label

2. Pills for staying awake

    a. Generally contain caffeine

    b. Should not be used to prolong wakefulness for more than an hour or two

G. Cosmetics

1. Skin Conditioners

    a. A dry skin will benefit from a simple oil, cream, or lotion

    b. Skin irritation may be reduced by common sense practices

2. Eye Cosmetics

    a. Should be used with care around eyes

    b. May carry microorganisms into the eyes

    c. Should be used with specific precautions

3. Deodorants and Antiperspirants

    a. Deodorants work against body odor

    b. Antiperspirants work against both wetness and body odor

    c. Body odor may best be controlled both by washing and by the use of a deodorant or antiperspirant

4. Other Deodorants

    a. Deodorants are also used for feet, vaginal hygiene, and body odors

    b. May come in form of dusts or powders

5. Products for acne

    a. Are not the answer to the problem

    b. Of more value are:

        (1) Proper diet

        (2) Cleanliness

        (3) Care by a physician

6. Suntans and Sunburns

    a. Both caused by ultraviolet rays

    b. Many lotions contain sunscreens

    c. Deep tanning may cause premature aging of the skin

    d. Skin care following sunbathing is important

7. Dandruff—treatment remains a matter of trial and error

8. Hair-removal products—chemical products must be used with great care

H. Safe Use of Cosmetics

    1. Read and follow all directions and warnings

    2. Wash your hands before applying a cosmetic

    3. Never borrow another person's cosmetics

    4. Never add saliva to a cosmetic

    5. See a physician immediately if an adverse reaction develops

IV. Selecting Safe Toys

    A. Care in buying and in parental supervision can reduce most toy injuries

    B. Toy should be too large to be swallowed, not have small detachable parts, not apt to break, not have sharp edges or points, not have exposed pins or nails, not be made of glass, labeled nontoxic, and not have parts which can pinch fingers

Questions for Review

1. What are the possible dangers in the self-diagnosis and self-treatment of minor symptoms?

2. In what circumstances should a physician be consulted?

3. Of what value is aspirin?

4. What precautions should be followed in using aspirin?

5. Why are drugstore remedies for colds of little value?

6. What are the potential hazards in the use of cold remedies?

7. What steps are important in preventing bad breath?

8. What is the basic cause of tooth decay?

9. Summarize the prevention of tooth decay.

10. What are common causes of constipation?

11. Why should laxatives never be self-prescribed?

12. What is a hemorrhoid?

13. What are the requirements for a good pair of sunglasses?

14. List the basic steps in caring for acne.

15. In addition to sunburn, what are the hazards in excessive exposure to the sun?

16. What are the basic types of dandruff and how is each best treated?

17. What precautions should be taken in the use of eye cosmetics?

18. Distinguish between the action of deodorants and antiperspirants.

19. List dangers to look for when buying toys for young children.

Chapter 4

CONSUMER PROTECTION

It has long been recognized that the consumer must have some protection against unscrupulous merchandizers of dangerous or worthless drugs and medical devices. *Caveat emptor,* "let the buyer beware," is still the working theme of many businesses. Few individual consumers possess the technical training, laboratory facilities, and money necessary to test health products for safety and effectiveness. The cost of testing a single drug may run into hundreds of thousands of dollars.

The average American possesses a low level of health information as confirmed by the results of the 1967 National Health Test. Well aware of this, advertisements for health products are directed to the emotions rather than to the intellect.

Due to the abuses consumers have suffered for decades, citizen groups have arisen which have made issues out of specific abuses and have demanded accountability of government regulatory agencies. Although these agencies were formed for the buyer's protection, they sometimes have made accommodation with the pressures from big business. This is an occasional criticism of regulatory agencies. Some feel that these agencies tend to reach working compromises with the businesses they regulate in order to correct gross abuses. In so doing, they may in time lose some of the sharpness of their regulatory functions. Under the emerging pressures of the nation's consumers, however, a kind of revival of purpose has been taking place on the part of some of these agencies. In this chapter some of these consumer protection efforts are detailed.

Semantics of Health Advertising

Alert businessmen know better than anyone else that the life-blood of their companies depends upon continued growth in sales. Expanding companies spare little in budget and talent to compete for the consumer's dollar. Some of the most attractive advertising copy is found in metropolitan newspapers, national magazines, and on oversized outdoor billboards. A particularly high advertising target is the highly vulnerable young adult and teenager.

Yet many of these glossy, full-color ads are calculatingly successful in their skillfully placed innuendos and half-truths. The ads feature beautiful people; sexual symbols and inferences are common. Following human sex instincts, such advertisers know all too well that a person with an obsession with sex has reduced sales resistance.

Of particular appeal are the advertisements for many of the nonprescription health products. Few other fields of writing offer such good examples of false implications, glittering generalities, and subtle misrepresentations. Government regulations clearly forbid the false advertising of health products. It is illegal, for example, to claim that a product can produce some result that in actuality it cannot produce, or to state that everyone can benefit from a product for which the majority of the population have no need.

Some of the most alluring advertising copy is found in cosmetic ads. The full-page color ads in the leading woman's magazines give some clue as to the earnings potential in the cosmetics market.

The ads, for example, tell us of (the italics are the authors'):

A cleansing lotion that destroys certain bacteria that *often* cause serious blemishes.

A moisture lotion that *replaces* and retains the moisture so vital to your skin.

A fingernail protection that makes your fingernails as *hard as nails*.

A line of cosmetics whose every product is a *scientific achievement*, irritant free and dermatologist tested.

A suntan lotion that gives the *"look of Hawaii."*

A waterproof eye shadow that won't run or streak through heat, humidity, or perspiration, yet is *incredibly natural looking*.

Shampoos and rinses that leave your hair naturally shiny, lustrous, easy to manage, and *free from tangling*.

A hair conditioner that works on the dry, dull parts of your hair *without* making the oily parts oilier.

No fingernail protection can make your fingernails as hard as nails; the Hawaiians would be hard pressed to describe to you the distinction between a suntanned appearance on the beaches of Waikiki and those of Laguna or Coney Island; no shampoo can keep your long hair free from tangling; any hair conditioner that adds oil to one part of your hair is adding oil to all parts of your hair; serious skin blemishes should be referred to a physician rather than treated with an over-the-counter product with no proof of effectiveness in countering skin infections.

Some health advertising is in open violation of the law. Advertising in this category is often for products such as hair growers, breast developers, and arthritis remedies. Government agencies can usually stop such frauds, though an ad may appear for some time before action can be taken, and many people can be deceived in the meantime.

More commonly, advertising copy is more cleverly written to stay (though just barely) within the letter of the law, while clearly violating the spirit of the law. Products advertised in this manner typically include remedies for headaches, hemorrhoids, anemia, coughs, colds, and the like. For example, in 1970 a product generally promoted for headaches (Excedrin) was advertised as being more effective in relieving pain than aspirin, but what was not stated in the ad was that the pain in the study cited was post-childbirth pain, not headache at all. Such advertising may deceive even an intelligent person and may be difficult or even impossible for government agencies to control.

In radio or TV advertising, voice inflection and tone can completely change the meaning that a straight reading of the same lines would convey. In printed advertising, the use of techniques such as large and small type size and deceptive ad layout can produce an ad which, while entirely within the law, is still grossly misleading.

Government Consumer Agencies

The Food and Drug Administration

The oldest federal government agency entirely concerned with consumer protection is the Food and Drug Administration (FDA), a branch of the U.S. Department of Health, Education, and Welfare. Since 1906, when the first Food and Drug Act was passed, this agency has attempted to protect the consumer against the dangers of contaminated food or hazardous or worthless drugs and medical devices. In the beginning, the FDA was mainly concerned with having dangerous products removed from the market. In 1938 the FDA received authority under the Food, Drug, and Cosmetic Act to inspect food plants and to require the clearance of new drugs for safety *before* they reach the market. Since 1962 additional steps have been taken to insure that drugs offered for sale are not only safe but effective as well.

The Federal Trade Commission

Created as a regulatory agency to proceed in the public interest against unfair methods of competition in commerce, the FTC has also acted upon deceptive practices as they concern the consumer of health products. It has acted against false and misleading advertising and selling practices that could adversely affect the health or safety of individuals. Typical actions involved hemorrhoid remedies that were claimed to shrink hemorrhoids so there would be no need for surgery; a vitamin-mineral preparation, aimed largely at older people, that was claimed to stimulate sexual vitality and activity; a drug product that would "prevent" or "cure" arthritis; and a book that claimed its suggestions were effective in preventing and treating cancer, heart disease, arthritis, and mental illness.

The Postal Service

The Postal Service, through its Postal Inspection System, works to prevent the mails from being used in schemes to defraud the public. The Postmaster General, through the Postal Inspection Service, is responsible for enforcing the postal laws. Postal Fraud statutes are found in two sections of the U.S. Code. Both prohibit the use of the mails to obtain money or property by means of false or fraudulent representations, pretenses, or promises. One provides felony penalties for mailings made in attempting to continue a fraud. The other allows the Service to refuse to deliver mail to the promoter, thus forcing him to shut down his mail-order operation.

One problem faced by the Postal Service in prosecuting and gaining convictions is that, according to the Mail Fraud Statute, *intent* to defraud must be proved. A second problem is that once people realize they have been duped by a scheme to relieve impotence or to increase bust size, they are often so embarrassed that it is difficult to persuade them to come forward and testify in court.

Private National Agencies

Several privately financed groups actively participate in consumer protection. The American Medical Association, through its Department of Investigation, Council on Foods, Council on Physical Medicine, and Department of Health Education, works to control fraudulent practices in various areas. *Today's Health,* a magazine published by the AMA, contains articles based on research done by its various departments and councils.

The Consumers Union is a nonprofit organization responsible for the monthly publication *Consumer Reports,* which reports evaluative research conducted through laboratory and use tests on many consumer products. The National Better Business Bureau is an organization promoting voluntary self-regulation of businesses in their advertising and sales representations.

State Departments of Consumer Affairs

Various individual states now have Departments of Consumer Affairs. In order to more completely develop accountability in the market place, they have been asking that consumers take a greater part in policing for misleading advertising. In California, for example, the law prohibits the dissemination of any advertisement which is false or deceptive, not just because it is unfair to the public, but because it is also a form of unfair competition which adversely affects ethical businesses.

The Department of Consumer Affairs in that state has issued a "consumer alert," asking those who have seen a newspaper, magazine, or direct-mail ad they consider to be untrue or misleading to send a copy of the ad to the department.

The request also applies to false and misleading labels. In the case of television or radio commercials, consumers are asked to make a note as to the date, time, content, and the channel or station on which the commercial ran. With billboards, they are instructed to make a note of the content as well as the date and location they saw it and the name of the billboard company involved. All such complaints are then to be sent to the Department of Consumer Affairs, Sacramento, California.

But despite the efforts of all these government and private agencies, worthless and even dangerous products continue to be available in drug stores and through mail-order sales. The mere fact that a drug or preparation is advertised appears to many consumers to constitute some warrant or justification of its safety and adequacy, if not its efficacy. If you have had any doubts about the merit of a particular product, check with a physician before you use it.

Consumer Laws

Two areas in which new consumer laws have been badly needed are in cosmetics and labeling. In both areas recently passed statutes are defining manufacturer accountability.

Laws Regulating Cosmetics

The cosmetics industry has been a long-standing area of lax FDA control. As of the beginning of 1976, consumers have the benefit of four new FDA regulations under the authority of the Fair Packaging and Labeling Act.

One requires that ingredients be listed on cosmetic labels, bringing consumers more information about what they buy and enabling them to make value comparisons among products. Another provides information on just who makes cosmetics; a third, on what goes into cosmetics; and a fourth, on what injuries or adverse reactions are being experienced by consumers. About 5000 different ingredients are used in cosmetics. With the new regulations all ingredients must be listed in order of predominance, with the ingredient present in the largest amount listed first, and so on down the list. Small packages must have attached tags or display cards providing sufficient room for all ingredients. Particularly helped are those consumers who are allergic to certain ingredients, such as copper powder, shark liver oil, dandelion root, or mistletoe. In order to protect trade secrets a manufacturer may list "and other ingredients" only upon permission granted by petition to the FDA.

According to the FDA Commissioner, this is the rationale for these regulations: "Ingredient labeling can be meaningful in preventing consumer deception by precluding product claims that are unreasonable in relation to the ingredients present and by providing consumers with additional information that can contribute to a knowledgeable judgment regarding the reasonableness of the price of the product. Furthermore, while ingredient identity may not be the sole determinant of a product's value to a consumer, it is one important criterion of a product's value in comparison with others. The presence of a substance to which a consumer is allergic or sensitive, for example, may render the product worthless to the consumer." People with allergies may know which ingredients they should avoid.

Consumers may also ask the manufacturer or the FDA what general purpose a certain ingredient serves. Without such information few would know, for instance, that *sodium laureth sulfate* is a cleansing and foaming agent used in shampoos. The FDA has now provided for a standardized name for each ingredient, so that the same ingredient bears the same name on each different product label. Lanolin oil goes by this name, rather than by one of 15 other names previously used among the trade for this ingredient.

Cosmetic manufacturers must identify themselves by filing name and address with the FDA. Under the second regulation the FDA asks that product formulas be filed. Under the third regulation the FDA asks the cosmetics industry to file data periodically on adverse reactions reported by consumers, helping determine any need for product reformulation or regulatory action. Consumers are asked to send complaints *directly* to the Food and Drug Administration, Division of Cosmetics Technology, Bureau of Foods, 211 C. St., S.W., Washington, D.C. 20004; instead of to the manufacturers.

More Effective Labeling

Thanks to the efforts of consumer advocates and certain government agencies, laws have been passed requiring manufacturers to put detailed labels on some goods. Two examples are *packaged food* and *cosmetics*.

Packaged Food

A new law being enforced as of January 1, 1975, requires that consumers be told, right on the label, what nutrients are in the food they buy. Under a standard format, the new food labels list the ingredients, what nutrients the food in the package will provide, and in what quantities. Uniform labeling enables consumers to compare the nutritional values of different foods.

Fig. 4.1 gives the standard format. The first line of the label will define the size of a serving or portion. The next line tells how many servings or portions are in the container. Then comes a breakdown of calories, protein, carbohydrates, and fat. Following total fat, an optional statement on the amounts of polyunsaturated and saturated fats may be reported. Next the manufacturer may state cholesterol content. Then comes the statement of protein, vitamin, and mineral content in percentages of the U.S. Recommended Daily Allowance (USRDA) for each.

Cosmetics

As of March 1974 all cosmetic labels printed must list ingredients such as specific colors (by government numbers—yellow #5, for example) and any possible irritants (lanolin, protein, coal tar). Certain coloring agents may be irritants to some users of those cosmetics.

Toys

Since late 1973 manufacturers of electrical toys have been required to state on every package: "Caution—Electrically operated product. Not rec-

NUTRITION INFORMATION
(Per Serving)
Serving Size = 8 Oz.
Servings per Container = 1

Calories	560	Fat (Percent of	
Protein	23 Grams	Calories 53%)	33 Grams
Carbohydrate	43 Grams	Polyunsaturated*	2 Grams
		Saturated	9 Grams
		Cholesterol*	
		(20 MG/100 G)	40 Milligrams
		Sodium	
		(365 MG/100 G)	830 Milligrams

PERCENTAGE OF U.S. RECOMMENDED DAILY ALLOWANCES
(USRDA)

Protein	35	Riboflavin	15
Vitamin A	35	Niacin	25
Vitamin C (Ascorbic Acid)	10	Calcium	2
Thiamine (Vitamin B₁)	15	Iron	25

*Information on fat and cholesterol content is provided for individulas who, on the advice of a physician, are modifying their total dietary intake of fat and cholesterol.

Figure 4.1 Standard Format for Nutrition Labeling.

ommended for children under eight years of age. As with all electric products, precautions should be observed during handling and use to prevent
electric shock."

Time must be given to manufacturers to switch to a new standard,
both in the printing of new labels and in the manufacture of the product
itself. Confusion tends to exist during this period. If a food manufacturer,
for example, had a large stockpile of canned fruit-drink labels (with a vitamin claim), he could continue to use them for a period of months (in this
case, through 1974). But any new labels ordered after January 1, 1974
must include nutrition information. As for the consumer, at the time of
purchase he must pick and choose among products to get the ones with
the new labels.

More information is still needed. Many foods do not have a complete
listing of the ingredients on the package; or when an ingredient is listed,
you only get half the necessary information. Ice cream products, for instance, don't require a list of ingredients such as coloring, binders, or
flavoring. Some food chains have started labeling ice cream voluntarily.
While the law requires that major ingredients be listed on certain food
packages, it does not require such a listing on certain "standardized foods"
or foods that must be made according to a government-regulated formula
(mayonnaise, ice cream, soft drinks). It would be convenient, however, to
know the ingredients of these if a person is allergic or sensitive to any of
them, such as to the cornstarch in ice cream.

Some consumers believe that medicines are automatically safe and
properly labeled just because they are medicines. This is not so. Although
the active ingredients in over-the-counter (patent medicine) products and
vitamins are listed, the inactive ingredients are not. These may be fillers,
binders, flavoring, and coloring. Some people have a sensitivity or intoler-
ance for certain colorings and other materials used as inactive ingredients
in medicines. For instance, lactose (a milk sugar), used as a filling in certain capsules, causes severe diarrhea in some people. A yellow food coloring (Food, Drug, and Cosmetics yellow #5) has induced asthma, hives,
and certain allergic reactions in some.

Medicines should have labels telling when they ought to be thrown
out. Some drugs lose their potency with age, and some even become dangerous when they deteriorate. Surely if photographic film and certain
perishable foods have expiration dates on them, medicines could also.

The use of a consumer package insert might be useful in providing
more consumer information on medicines. The FDA is testing such an
insert for the recently approved birth-control preparations DES (the
"morning after" pill) and Depo Provera (the three-month contraceptive
injection). The inserts frankly tell some facts on the potential dangers of
these drugs. In this manner the consumer can make a more intelligent
choice of the benefits versus the risks of the various birth-control devices
and drugs. Such inserts may well be useful for other drugs, particularly

those to be taken over a longer period when a patient might not be seeing a physician regularly.

All consumers need to take more time to read labels. Hopefully, with the new legislation and through the efforts of consumer advocates, there will be increasing reason to expand the effort.

Consumer Action

What steps can I as a consumer take to support consumer action? One is to support consumer councils, such as in the area of secret prescription pricing. A second area of action is in filing personal complaints over product violations to the proper government agency.

Secret Prescription Pricing

It has been customary in the U.S. for an ill person to receive a scribbled prescription from the physician which is taken to any pharmacy to be filled without regard to price. Consumer advocates, legislators, and federal agencies are now openly challenging this time-honored practice. Why, if the cost of virtually every other product is advertised somewhere, shouldn't the customer know what he or she will have to pay for a prescription?

Each year Americans have filled an estimated 1.5 billion prescriptions at an average price of a little over $4.00 per prescription. While perhaps insignificant to the generally well individual, this can be a heavy expense to the elderly and to patients with long-term illness. It is possible for such patients to pay hundreds of dollars extra over a period of years if they buy through a pharmacy that charges two or three times as much as a lower-priced one. In a study by the Boston Consumers' Council, a south side pharmacy charged $8 for the antibiotic Achromycin, while one on the north side charged $2.60 for the same amount of the same drug. Many pharmacies will not quote a price over the phone or at the counter until the prescription is ready for purchase. In many states there are existing laws prohibiting the advertising of prescription drug pricing; some states even have restrictions that actually prevent pharmacists from telling the elderly that a discount is available to them. While some state courts have declared unconstitutional the state laws that bar the advertising of prescription drugs, similar restrictions have been upheld by courts in other states. The state of Vermont requires, on the other hand, that pharmacies must post the 100 most commonly prescribed drugs and their current selling prices.

There are several reasons why drug prices may vary. The first is that druggists keep inaccurate stock records (their wholesale drug costs). Another is in the way pharmacists set prices. One method commonly used by the pharmacist is to set his retail price by applying a formula using the wholesale cost to him and then setting a percentage of profit. Another method is the professional fee method in which the pharmacist estimates how much he needs to pay for overhead expenses and make a profit and then computes a specific fee for dispensing prescriptions. The customer's cost then becomes the fee plus the wholesale cost of the drug. The advantage here is that since the fee is identical for all prescriptions, the pharmacist has no reason to pick a costlier brand if the physician's prescription gives him that option. A third method used by some pharmacists is a flexible arrangement in which the charge depends upon the time and skill needed to fill the prescription.

Opponents to advertising contend that posting of prices can cover only a hundred or so of the several thousand items a pharmacy may have in stock, and that the druggist may lower his prices on the advertised prices but make it up on the unlisted prices. Others contend that drugs are simply not commodities like groceries or tires and that prescription posting puts undue emphasis on price.

In any event, there are several steps any person can take to keep his or her drug prices down.

1. Talk prescription prices over with your physician. You should expect the physician to have some idea what prescription medicines cost patients and to direct you to drug stores that charge the lowest price for the best quality drug.

2. Ask your physician to write down the name, quantity, and strength of your medication on a slip of paper separate from the prescription. Then check and compare prices.

3. If you are taking medication for a long term illness, know that pills and capsules usually cost less in quantities of 100 or 500. Larger volumes of pills, if needed for the illness, may be proper for you if the particular pill doesn't become unstable quickly. Get your physician to prescribe by the generic, or chemical name, rather than by the brand name.

4. Find out from the pharmacist if that particular drug store provides a discount for the elderly.

5. Take into account the pharmacy's service, as well as its price. Extra service and convenience may more than offset the extra cost.

Guidelines for Filing Consumer Complaints

When the top of your dining room table is ruined by the furniture polish, when the canned tuna smells tainted, or when a skin conditioner causes a rash, there is more to do than throw the product away and vow to buy a different brand the next time. You can, and should, report complaints to the proper government agency. The problem lies in knowing how and to whom to register a complaint.

Here are some steps for the consumer to follow before filing a complaint, as well as some instruction on how and where to report such a complaint.

Before You Report

Before a consumer reports violations or hazards, the following questions should be asked:

Have I used the product as labeled?
Did I follow the instructions carefully?
Did an allergy contribute toward the bad effect?
Was the product old when I opened it?

Make sure all these factors have been taken into consideration first to confirm that the complaint lies with the product, not the consumer's misuse of it.

How to Report

Report the complaint as soon as possible. Give your name, address, telephone number, and directions on how to get to your home or place of business. Clearly state the complaint. Describe in as much detail as possible the label of the product. Give any date or code marks that appear on the container (with canned goods these are usually stamped or embossed on the lid of the can). Give the name and address of the store where the article was bought and the date of purchase. Save whatever remains of the product or the empty container for your physician's guidance or possible examination by the FDA. Retain any unopened containers of the product you bought at the same time. If an injury is involved, see your physician at once. Report the suspect product to the manufacturer, packer, or distributor shown on the label, and to the store where you bought it.

Where to Report

There are basically 10 agencies with jurisdiction over such products that one can turn to with a complaint. These agencies and their areas of responsibility include:

Food and Drug Administration: drugs and medicines (human and veterinary); medical devices; cosmetics; and medical preparations made from living organisms and their products.

Federal Trade Commission: suspected false advertising.

Consumer Product Safety Commission: toys; laundry, cleaning, and polishing products; home repair and paint products; hobbyist items; and automotive fluids.

U.S. Department of Agriculture: meat and poultry products.

The Postal Service: mail order frauds and unsolicited products by mail.

U.S. Department of Justice, Bureau of Narcotics and Dangerous Drugs: illegal sale of narcotics or dangerous drugs (such as stimulants, depressants, and hallucinogens).

Environmental Protection Agency: pesticides; air and water pollution.

State Health Department: products made and sold exclusively within your state.

State Board of Pharmacy: dispensing practices of pharmacies and drug prices.

Poison Control Centers: accidental poisonings.

Since many of the health complaints are filed with the Food and Drug Administration, here are special instructions for filing complaints with the FDA. The complaint may be filed in writing or by phone to the nearest FDA field office or resident inspection station. The FDA has 10 regional offices, 19 district offices, and 97 resident inspection stations throughout the United States. In cities with no FDA office or inspection station, the address and phone number of the nearest FDA office may be found in the telephone directory under U.S. Government, Department of Health, Education, and Welfare, Food and Drug Administration. A consumer may also write directly to FDA headquarters: *Food and Drug Administration, 5600 Fishers Lane, Rockville, Maryland 20852.*

Summary

I. Semantics of Health Advertising

    A. Advertising is the life-blood of expanding companies

    B. Advertisements often contain false implications, innuendoes, generalities, and half-truths

    C. Important to examime them critically and objectively

II. Government Consumer Agencies

    A. Food and Drug Administration (FDA)

    B. Federal Trade Commission (FTC)

    C. Postal Service

    D. Private National Agencies

        1. American Medical Association

        2. Consumers Union

        3. National Better Business Bureau

    E. State Departments of Consumer Affairs

III. Consumer Laws—two major new laws

    A. Laws Regulating Cosmetics—four new regulations

        1. Ingredients must be listed on cosmetic labels

        2. Information must be provided to the FDA on who makes cosmetics

        3. What goes into cosmetics must be made known

        4. Injuries or adverse reactions experienced by consumers must be made public to the FDA

    B. More Effective Labeling

        1. Food—must list nutritional values such as calories, protein, fat content, carbohydrates, vitamins, and minerals

        2. Cosmetics—(see above)

        3. Toys—must identify electrically operated toys; not recommended for children under eight years of age

IV. Consumer Action—What Can Consumer Do?

    A. Support consumer councils, such as in the area of secret prescription pricing

    B. File personal complaints over product violations to:

        1. FDA

        2. FTC

        3. Consumer Product Safety Commission

        4. U.S. Department of Agriculture

        5. Postal Service

        6. U.S. Department of Justice

        7. Environmental Protection Agency

        8. State Health Department

        9. State Board of Pharmacy

        10. Poison Control Centers

Questions for Review

1. What is the meaning of *caveat emptor?*

2. What do the initials FDA and FTC stand for and what is the work of each agency?

3. Give the names of some private national agencies engaged in consumer protection.

4. In what four ways do new FDA regulations place greater responsibility on the cosmetics industry?

5. On what three kinds of goods must new detailed labels be affixed?

6. What steps can a person take to help keep drug prices down?

7. In what way did the Boston Consumer Council effect action against secret drug pricing?

8. What three questions should you answer before you file a consumer complaint?

9. How should a person go about filing a complaint?

10. Give six government agencies concerned with consumer products and the products over which each has jurisdiction.

Chapter 5
QUACKERY

The colorful traveling medicine show may be a thing of the past, but medical quackery is still very much a part of the modern scene. Today's quack is much more sophisticated than was the "snake oil" salesman of the past, but his goal is still the same—to separate the suckers from their money. The quack seems to be sincerely interested in a person's health, but the real interest is in making money—lots of money. The cost of medical quackery in the United States today is estimated at between one and two *billion* dollars a year. Modern quackery takes several common forms: it may involve a direct "doctor-patient" relationship, the mail-order or house-to-house sale of worthless products, or the sale in drug or "health food" stores of products that cannot do what is claimed of them.

Who Are the Quacks?

A *quack* may be defined as a boastful pretender to medical skill, who promises medical benefits which he cannot deliver. The quack may attempt to go beyond the limits of medical science or the limits of his or her own training.

Your own mental image of a quack may be that of an odd- or sinister-looking individual, but by actual appearance it is impossible to tell a quack from an ethical physician. Any quack may be wearing a conservative business suit or a white medical-type coat. His or her personality is likely to be friendly, self-confident, and confidence-inspiring. You just "know" this person is well qualified.

Some quacks are well-intentioned persons who feel they have something to contribute to the health and well-being of other people; yet they are actually ignorant of the basic principles of health and nutrition. Quacks are sometimes owners or operators of, or employees in, health food stores dispensing unaccurate and poorly founded nutritional and/or health information. While well intentioned, such diagnosing of health and nutritional problems can be as dangerous for the unwary consumer as the overt actions of the most ill-intentioned and sinister quack.

Quacks have various kinds of training. Once in a great while a licensed medical physician enters into an area of quackery. A few large-selling books have been written by such doctors. Much more common is the quack who has had more limited medical training, perhaps in chiropractic or naturopathic (a drugless therapy, making use of air, light, water, heat, massage, and other physical forces) methods. Many convicted quacks show no record of any formal higher education. College degrees and transcripts are obtainable from print shops and "diploma mill" colleges. The word "Doctor" in front of a name or the degrees after a name may mean nothing. Sometimes the quack is not an individual at all but a corporation which makes false claims for its products. And, of course, *self-treatment is quackery* if an individual tries to diagnose and treat a serious illness by himself.

Quackery often involves the sale or application of a *nostrum,* a cure-all drug or machine. Any drug or machine for which the producer makes exaggerated claims can be called a nostrum.

Who Turns to Quackery?

All kinds of people become the victims of quacks—the old and the young, the rich and the poor, and everyone in-between. But quacks do seem to prey particularly upon the extremes—the young, the elderly, the very rich, and the very poor.

The young person often becomes the victim of mail-order quackery. There are many deceptive advertisements in certain of the magazines that appeal to young people. The products offered promise good looks, popularity, and sex appeal. There are products which are claimed to help gain weight, lose weight, build muscles, enlarge the breasts, and cure acne. Seldom are these products of any real value.

Elderly people find appeal in products that promise to renew their lost youth and vigor. They often waste their limited money on treatments and products which claim to relieve arthritis, impotency, prostate conditions, gray hair, baldness, and "tired blood," when, in fact, they may produce no such result. The nutrition quack caters to elderly people who are led to believe that all their aches and pains can disappear through the use of certain food products or food supplements. In addition, the elderly are attracted to so-called "clinics" and "health ranches" which claim cures for various chronic diseases through chiropractic, fad diets, and other limited methods.

Quacks are interested in the rich simply because they have money. The poor are receptive to quackery because good medical services are often scarce in low-income areas; the cost of ethical care may seem prohibitive; and the poorly educated may not even realize the difference between ethical medicine and quackery.

Fear, Ignorance, and Gullibility

Much quackery preys upon *fear*. Anyone who has been told by a physician that he or she has an incurable disease lives in fear—fear of death, fear of pain, fear of surgery, fear of the unknown. Such a person may grasp at any straw of hope offered by the quack, no matter how unscientific or expensive the treatment may be. Sometimes fear keeps a person from seeking an ethical physician in the first place. Afraid of surgery, a person may turn instead to a quack who promises a cure without surgery. Sometimes a quack must create fear where none exists. The quack may, for example, tell a perfectly healthy person that he or she has a serious disease and then recommend an expensive series of worthless treatments for the nonexistent disorder. The constant fear of imminent health disaster may lead some persons to continuous self-treatment, an often bizarre regiment of self-administered "preventive medicine."

Ignorance and gullibility are strong allies of the quack. Millions of people are almost unbelievably gullible. These people unquestioningly accept almost anything they hear as truth, and anything they read is accepted as absolute gospel. A quack can make sales talks and literature seem entirely believable to such people. Even well-educated people who should know better often fall for quack schemes because no one can be completely knowledgeable in all areas. Most people lack sufficient medical background to know if what they've been told is reasonable or not; yet they have just enough medical background to enable them to recognize a few names of diseases or medications. For this reason quackery follows right on the coattails of science.

Major Types of Quackery Today

Cancer Quackery

Despite the intensive efforts of government agencies to control cancer quackery, millions of dollars are still being spent every year for worthless cancer treatments. Cancer quackery is one of the most tragic of all rackets because many persons with early, curable cancers waste vital time waiting for a worthless remedy to cure their cancer. By the time they seek ethical treatment, their cancers have often progressed to an incurable stage.

Early treatment by an ethical physician using standard methods can often result in the complete cure of cancer today.

Examples of cases in which cancer patients have lost valuable time following quacks are numerous. Here are a couple of case histories.

Case 1. The lady was a legal secretary, age 42. Three years earlier she had undergone a bilateral mastectomy (removal of both breasts). For the past eight months she had felt quite fatigued and upon the recommendation of a friend, she made an appointment for an examination by a physician new to her. The physician took no usual tests (blood pressure, body temperature, etc.) but said he was able to diagnose patients by merely *looking* at them. He suspected a staphylococcus infection in the mouth (the patient had nine teeth pulled, although there were no signs of visible decay) and treated her with antibiotics (which he supplied) and vitamin B shots. He set up a weekly appointment for eight months at $12 a visit. Every two weeks he gave the patient antibiotics for an additional charge of $26 each time (he assured her his dispensing of the antibiotics amounted to a discount to her because of the "good price he got on them").

The physician employed no nurse. He "didn't want anyone interfering with him and the patient"—he wanted direct contact. He expected patients to pay for each office call immediately—in cash. He "couldn't be bothered with Blue Cross, or any other form of health insurance." The physician accepted patients *only* on the recommendation of other patients.

The physician instructed the patient to quit work when the treatment started, and she went on disability—although in the past she had resumed working after a leave from her job for the mastectomy. She became concerned when she didn't appear to recover from her intense fatigue. Out of desperation she went to a nearby clinic, where those in charge insisted she leave her "cancer physician" immediately and seek therapy in a reputable tumor clinic. But for admission she needed a statement of referral from her present physician. Her "cancer physician" refused referral when requested. She was finally admitted to the tumor clinic through special arrangements. Immediate examination confirmed cancer of the spine and chest, and suspected leukemia.

At the date of this writing, the "cancer physician" is still practicing at the same location. He is listed in the telephone directory as a medical doctor specializing in neuropsychiatry and endocrinology.

Case 2. In this case, a chiropractor was ultimately convicted of second degree murder in the death of a child he had promised to cure of cancer, and he is now serving a term of five years to life imprisonment. The patient (later victim) was an eight-year-old whose mother became concerned over a slight swelling over her daughter's left eye. She was taken to UCLA Medical Center, where exploratory surgery revealed a tumorous mass in the left orbit, which was diagnosed as an extremely malignant and fast-growing form of cancer. An examination also revealed that there was no evidence of the spread of the cancer to any other part of her body. The parents were told that it was necessary to remove the eye and all of the surrounding tissue in the eye orbit. The parents consented to the surgery, but before it could be performed, they met a couple who claimed their own son had been cured of a brain tumor without surgery by the chiropractor. Consulted by phone, he gave them absolute assurances he could help their daughter (without having seen the child or her medical records). His diagnosis of the cause of the cancer was a "chemical imbalance" which surgery would only make worse. Upon his insistence, the daughter was taken out of the UCLA hospital where, he claimed, they would only use her as a guinea pig and "get their money." His own fee—$500 in advance plus $200 to $300 a month for medicine! The daughter was immediately examined by the chiropractor and diagnosed as having hypochronic anemia, inflammation of the gall bladder, possible kidney disease, hyperthyroidism, but no mention of cancer. Treatment included 124 pills (vitamins, food supplements, laxatives) daily, 150 drops of an iodine solution in a glass of water each hour for 11 hours a day, a two-quart enema every other day, daily musculo-skeletal adjustments in his office, and instructions for the parents to daily manipulate the ball of the daughter's foot with sufficient pressure to cause her to cry (which the parents refused to do).

After over three weeks of "care," the tumor had enlarged to the size of a tennis ball and had pushed the eye out of the socket and down along the nose. The parents discharged the chiropractor and brought the daughter back to UCLA, where her condition was now recognized as hopeless. Four months later she died.[1]

Case 3. A decade ago a mysterious cancer drug called Krebiozen was exposed. Suddenly "discovered" by a Yugoslavian exile physician, it was brought from South America to Illinois, where it won the support of an internationally known physiologist, who was also at the time the vice president of the University of Illinois. Although the drug was available in Illinois, the federal government refused to allow it to be sold interstate until it was shown to be safe and efficacious. Sample analyses varied from batch to batch, as well as did the claims of its supporters. It was eventually shown to consist of creatine (a substance naturally found in the body in far greater concentrations than those of the drug) dissolved in mineral oil. Most disturbing was that then U.S. Senators Javits, Case, and Douglas argued on the floor of the U.S. Senate to have the normal FDA testing requirements for new drugs waived so that the Krebiozen Foundation could make this marvelous drug available immediately to dying cancer patients. After Krebiozen was rejected by the National Cancer Institute, the American Cancer Society, and the Federal Drug Administration, the sale of the drug in the state of Illinois was finally terminated. The exile physician was later charged with tax fraud by the IRS, indicted, and convicted on that charge.

---

[1] The American Cancer Society *Volunteer* 16:2 (1970).

The cancer quack often claims to use an effective treatment which is exclusively his and unavailable to other physicians; or he or she claims that regular doctors don't want to use effective cures for cancer because it would hurt their business. These claims are, of course, ridiculous. If these remedies were effective, physicians and their families would take advantage of them when faced with a diagnosis of cancer. Effective medical treatments cannot be kept exclusive in the United States, and ethical doctors certainly do not need dying cancer patients in order to stay busy. There are very few ethical doctors in this country who are not already busier than they would like to be.

A strong ally of the cancer quack is the fear of surgery felt by many people. The quack always promises a cure without surgery, but in ethical medicine, surgery is one of the most important treatments for most kinds of cancer.

Arthritis Quackery

Arthritis, sometimes called rheumatism, is an inflammation of the joints. Millions of people suffer from some degree of arthritis, with great pain and crippling in extreme cases. Ethical medicine can offer a real cure for only a few of the many types of arthritis. About half of all arthritis sufferers are therefore led to try quack remedies, at a cost of about a quarter of a billion dollars a year.

Some types of arthritis periodically come and go, even without treatment; thus, quack remedies are often given credit for curing cases of arthritis which would have gone away even if nothing had been done. With arthritis, as well as any other disease, the ethical physician can still be relied upon to offer the most effective, up-to-date treatment available.

Food Quackery

Food quackery is a big business. Over *ten million* Americans are today living in the shadow of confusion cast by the food faddists and "health food" quacks. These unfortunate people are encouraged to follow expensive, complicated, and often unpleasant diets. Rather than being better fed as a result, they are actually more likely to suffer from nutritional deficiency than those who eat ordinary diets, following the simple rules of basic nutrition.

Myths about Foods

Food quackery products are sold in several ways. They are often featured in "health food" stores, sold by door-to-door salespersons, advertised for mail-order sale, and promoted in "health" lectures. Regardless of the sales approach used, the food quack makes use of scare tactics, calculated to frighten people into buying these products. Almost all operators in this field make use of certain modern myths. Each of these myths may contain some elements of truth, but the conclusions drawn by the quack are not supported by scientific evidence. The following are some of these myths:

1. *Myth that all disease is due to a faulty diet.* Of course, deficiency diseases such as scurvy are entirely the result of poor diet, and one's resistance to many infectious diseases is lower when diet is poor. But no known diet can protect a person from all infectious diseases or from cancer, as is claimed for certain nutrition products.

2. *Myth of the indispensable food product.* Salespersons often represent their products as being the only source of a vital food substance and imply that maximum good health is possible only if their products are used. The truth is that every substance known to be important in nutrition is available from a variety of common grocery-store foods. The salesperson will often counter this fact by saying that his or her product contains some substance not yet known to science. However, there is absolutely no basis for such a claim.

3. *Myths about soil depletion.* Another common story is that years of farming the same land has removed vital substances from the soil and that the food produced is therefore deficient. While it is true that an iodine deficiency in the soil is reflected in the food produced, bad effects from iodine deficiency are rare today because most people do receive adequate iodine from their food and from iodized salt. If any other mineral is lacking from the soil, the result is a reduced quantity of the crop, but the food's nutritional quality is not damaged.

4. *Myths about "organic" or "natural" foods.* Almost every product sold as a "health food" or food supplement is advertised as being "organic" or "natural," or both. The word "organic" can properly be defined in two ways: it may mean "derived from living organisms" or "based on atoms of carbon." All foods, even those in the grocery store, fit both definitions of the word. The word "organic" is usually used in the "health food" business to imply that food has been grown with manure instead of commercial fertilizers. The claim is made that food grown with commercial (chemical) fertilizer is inferior to that grown with manure. The truth is that a plant can only absorb certain simple inorganic nutrients from the soil. If manure or other organic matter is applied as fertilizer, the organic compounds present must break down to the same inorganic compounds contained in commercial fertilizers before any absorption into the roots of the plant can take place.

A similar claim is that the synthetically produced vitamins are inferior to naturally occurring vitamins. This statement is usually made by salespersons of higher-priced products to indicate their product's superiority over lower-priced synthetic products. The truth is that man-made vitamins are chemically identical to naturally occurring vitamins. They are absorbed into the body in the same way and function in exactly the same manner.

The very word "chemical" is often used in a disparaging manner by salespersons who apparently do not know, or choose to ignore, the fact, that all food is merely a mixture of chemicals. These salespersons tell us that grocery-store foods are made poisonous by chemical additives. The truth is that the Food and Drug Administration rigidly controls the use of food additives, so that in the amounts used they are perfectly safe. The withdrawal of cyclamates from the market serves to illustrate this protection.

5. *Myths about vitamins.* Recently there have been claims of unusual therapeutic effect for a host of conditions through the use of huge doses of vitamins E, B, and C. No claims have been more spectacular than those made for vitamin E. Because of the widespread confusion over contradictory reports on this vitamin, the National Academy of Sciences National Research Council has issued a public statement regarding the misinformation.

The list of ailments claimed to be relieved by vitamin E is staggering. It includes most non-infectious diseases such as heart disease, sterility, muscular weakness, cancer, ulcers, skin diseases, burns, and shortness of breath. Beyond this, vitamin E has been claimed to promote physical endurance, enhance sexual potency, prevent heart attacks, protect against the health-related aspects of air pollution, and slow the aging process and alleviate its accompanying ailments.

Where do claims of such "miraculous cures" come from? Where do people get such ideas? To begin with, it is a fact that small amounts of vitamin E are necessary for normal life; but notions as to its miraculous powers come from unscientific interpretation of certain laboratory research. Take, for instance, the sterility-prevention claims. While vitamin E has been shown in experiments (with vitamin E deficient rats) to prevent sterility, and also natural abortion, studies with humans have failed to produce any evidence whatsoever that additional vitamin E does anything of the kind in people. Its reproductive effect was shown only in laboratory animals when they had been purposely deprived of vitamin E for long periods of time. The same thing happened regarding muscular weakness studies in animals, but according to the Council, studies have produced no evidence that vitamin E has any effect on muscular dystrophy in humans.

The story was repeated in claims regarding heart disease and vitamin E. Large doses have been advocated for angina pectoris, coronary occlusion, congestive heart failure, thrombophlebitis, and thromboembolism. Although the dosage recommended by the NRC for adults is 30 units (1 mg. of synthetic vitamin E supplies one international unit) per day, hundreds of thousands of persons have been consuming up to one gram a day (about 35 times the daily requirement). While insufficient amounts of vitamin E cause serious heart diseases in cows, sheep, and other grass eaters, no heart disease has ever been related to a vitamin E deficiency in man. To date, extensive tests have failed to demonstrate any therapeutic benefit from supplemental vitamin E.

Why does there appear to be some connection between a vitamin E deficiency and these various conditions in animals where there isn't in humans? The reason, according to the Council, is that vitamin E deficiency is extraordinarily rare among Americans on an average diet. An ample supply of the vitamin is found in substantial amounts in the foods we eat every day. The chief sources of vitamin E in the diet are wheat germ oil and other vegetable oils and vegetables, especially lettuce. Infants and children with intestinal conditions that prevent them from absorbing nutrients properly are the individuals most likely to have a vitamin E deficiency. About the only people short on vitamin E are premature infants and people suffering from conditions that interfere with digestion or absorption of fats. Both of these groups should be, and usually are, under the care of a physician.

For the large majority of people, the NRC advises, "self medication with vitamin E in the hope that a more or less serious condition will be alleviated may be hazardous, especially when appropriate diagnosis and treatment may thereby be delayed or avoided."

Such are the myths that have fueled the vitamin E craze and lined with gold the pockets of the manufacturers of this vitamin.

6. *Myths about food processing.* The food quack exaggerates the loss of food value through modern food processing methods. Such a person may even say that we are slowly starving to death as a result. Although some loss definitely does occur, it is minor in comparison with the benefit we receive from modern food technology. Today's processing methods are often less destructive to vitamins than were the methods used in the past. Highly nutritious "processed" fruits, vegetables, and meats are now available throughout the year, rather than just during limited seasons. The vitamin loss seldom exceeds 25 percent and is generally much less than that. Although fresh, unprocessed food is preferable, processed food is not as bad as food faddists claim.

One of the most unfortunate targets of attacks by food faddists has been white bread. According to Dr. Olaf Mickelsen, president of the American Institute of Nutrition and professor of human nutrition and foods and of biochemistry at Michigan State University, white bread still has a great deal to offer. A slice of enriched white bread contains only about 60 calories. A pat of butter doubles the calorie count; a slice of cheddar adds another 150 calories. Experiments at the university indicate that bread can serve most of the protein needs of a person.

According to the Department of Foods and Nutrition of the American Medical Association, flour enrichment was never meant to restore nutrients lost in milling but rather was designed to help correct nutritional deficiencies common 30 years ago. Bleaching flour ages it and makes it look whiter rather than destroying nutrients. The whitening is in response to consumer demands. Furthermore, aging improves flour's baking quality. Unbleached flour that has been aged is slightly golden in color but doesn't differ significantly from bleached flour in nutritional quality. Chemical bleaching now replaces the older, costlier method of storing and turning flour in warehouses for long periods to speed oxidation. Contrary to fad-dists' claims, there are only minor nutritional differences between whole wheat and enriched white bread. Ordinary bakers' white bread contains only about 3.5% fat, much of which is polyunsaturated because it comes from wheat oils. It is also a low-cholesterol product unless the baker adds eggs and whole milk.

Results of Food Quackery

The most surprising result of this over-concern with nutrition is that it may not result in a balanced diet. Too often the quack or faddist concentrates on a few specific food elements and ignores others, perhaps to the point of deficiency. There may even be excessive amounts of certain nutrients, especially the fat-soluble vitamins, such as A and D, which can accumu-late in the body to harmful levels.

The most dangerous medical result of food quackery is that diet ther-apy often delays necessary medical treatment of serious disorders. Self-diagnosis and self-treatment are some of the most dangerous forms of quackery. Describing symptoms to a food supplement salesperson or drugstore clerk, who then "prescribes" various products as remedies, is equally dangerous. There are many serious physical disorders which may prove fatal without prompt medical treatment.

"Reduce Without Dieting"

One out of every four Americans tries to lose weight each year. These fifty million people provide a ready market for any product which promises an easy way to lose weight without unpleasant dieting. Unfortunately, there is no "easy" way to lose weight. Weight can only be lost by eating less and/or by increasing activity level. Some of the schemes offered include:

1. *Nonprescription pills.* Most reducing pills sold without a prescrip-tion are too weak to be of any real value. If a pill is strong enough to help in weight loss, it should be used only under medical direction.

2. *Spot reducing.* It is absolutely impossible to control fat loss from a specific part of the body. At best, muscle tone can be improved to give a slimmer appearance.

3. *Vibrators.* Fat cannot be vibrated off.

4. *Massaging devices.* Neither can it be massaged away.

5. *Reducing creams.* These have absolutely no effect.

Bust Development

Due to our national obsession with breasts, some women have come to feel sexually inadequate or self-conscious because of their small breasts. The size of the breasts is determined by hormone levels and hereditary factors. The "girlie" magazines, movies, and other entertainment forms have contributed to an exaggerated idea of ideal breast size, since they feature those few women with unusually large breast development.

Many schemes for breast development are offered to the "flat" woman. Unfortunately, most of these are ineffective and some are actually harmful. They include:

1. *Special exercises.* Of all the plans offered, special exercises offer the most hope of a larger-appearing bust line without danger. Exercises will *not* increase the size of the breasts, but they can increase the development of the chest muscles, giving the appearance of greater breast development. They will *not,* as some gyms and exercise machine producers advertise, increase the bra size "from 32A to 36D."

2. *Special diets.* Nothing, outside of a normal balanced diet, can be eaten that will contribute to breast development.

3. *Breast development creams.* No cream applied to the breasts can safely increase their size. If a product contains hormones, its use could be dangerous without adequate medical supervision.

4. *Silicone implants and injections.* National magazines have given much publicity to silicone as a means of increasing breast size. Medical authorities and the Food and Drug Administration strongly condemn this method of enlarging the breasts. The dangers inherent in these procedures far outweigh any possible benefits.

The "flat" woman should realize that there is no relationship between breast size and sexual adequacy or femininity. While large breasts might be of value to a "topless" dancer, they are of no particular value in everyday life. In fact, large breasts are not even important for success in nursing a baby. Thus, a woman should accept her figure as it is and save her anxieties for more important problems.

Some Specific Examples of Quackery

The following specific examples of quackery have been selected from recent issues of *FDA Papers,* an official publication of the Food and Drug Administration. They should serve to illustrate the types of fraud and deception to which the public is being subjected today.

Mail Fraud Cases Reported by the U.S. Postal Service

"Advertising and sale by mail of U.S. Women's Ski Team Diet, represented to be effective in causing a weight loss of 20 pounds in 2 weeks" (November 1973).

"Representations by mail that diagnosis of medical ailments can be made on the basis of a saliva test submitted through the mail" (January 1974).

"Solicitations and sale through the mail of 'Marula Pips,' 'Marula Pip Tea Bags,' and 'Marula Concentrate,' represented to be effective remedies for male sexual impotence and female frigidity" (January 1973).

"Advertising and sale by mail of 'Passiflora' liquid, represented as one of the most sought-after offerings for satisfying marital relations" (March 1973).

"Advertising and sale through the mails of 'Eat-Well' tablets, represented as enabling an obese person to reduce without dieting" (February 1973).

"Solicitations and sale by mail of 'European Love Drops 5,' represented as an effective aphrodisiac or sexual stimulant" (April 1973).

"Advertising and sale by mail of 'H-3' tablets, represented to be an effective cure for arthritis and 'mental and nervous confusion'" (April 1973).

"Advertising and sale by mail of 'La Placenta,' represented to be effective as a sex stimulant, bust developer, and wrinkle remover" (March 1973).

"Advertising and sale by mail of a diet called 'Magic Plan,' represented to enable persons to lose 16 pounds in 4 days, 22 pounds in a week, or 37 pounds in a month" (December 1973).

Products Seized by the Food and Drug Administration

Product (date)	Charge
Electromagnetic energy generator (9/2/72)	False and misleading claims for infections, fractures, bone and tissue healing, bursitis, arthritis, low back pain, blood flow to peripheral areas, and sinusitis.
Candy bars (12/5/72)	False and misleading representations that vitamin E provided energy and stamina, and that such a candy bar was necessary and useful in supplementing the diet with vitamin E.
Battery-operated vibrator pads for face, throat, and breasts, and pink "firming" cream (5/31/72)	False and misleading claims to firm the body; provide a firmer, healthier, more attractive appearance; renew the firmness of youth in a woman's face, chin, and breasts; restore and build muscles and muscle elasticity; create better circulation; tighten and firm soft and sagging skin tissues, saggy breasts, double chins, and flabby jaws; tone the muscle fibers that support the breasts and develop and strengthen these muscles to return them to their natural shape and firmness.
Herb tablets (7/24/72)	False and misleading claims as a laxative and poultice for bladder stones, common cold, tuberculosis, high fever, dysentery, rattlesnake bite, dandruff, body odor, and "weakness-laziness."

"Sound sleep" plastic filled pillows containing magnets (4/17/73)

False and misleading claims for insomnia, hyperactive children, easing tension and nervous tension, create a magnetic field inside the pillow which neutralized anxiety, and producing electrical impulses in the nerve center which caused natural sleep.

Bubble gum (9/15/71)

In violation of the Fair Packaging and Labeling Act, since the principal display panel area lacked any quantity of contents declaration.

Rice (5/25/73)

Contained rodent filth and was held under insanitary conditions.

Aspirin tablets for pets (7/13/72)

False and misleading claims for use to calm and relieve nervousness, cold symptoms, and aches and pains generally in pets, and to relieve and prevent motion sickness from plane, train, or automobile travel.

Egg shampoo (5/22/72)

False and misleading claims; not in conformity with the Fair Packaging and Labeling Act.

Squeeze toys (5/10/72)

Articles were banned as being hazardous substances intended for use by children and presenting mechanical hazards by reason of the potential of the exposed squeaker attachments for being ingested and causing asphyxiation.

Seasonings, bouillon, and other special dietary foods (9/3/70)

False and misleading claims that the article would build teeth; provide instant energy, a full meal, all nutrients needed by the body, and a balance of minerals; and that balanced natural food was our only real medicine.

Saltine crackers (5/2/72)

Article contained the nonconforming food additive Ronnel, a pesticide chemical, and the article had been prepared, packed, and held under insanitary conditions whereby it may have been rendered injurious to health.

Cough syrup for dogs (5/26/71)

Labeling contained false and misleading claims for relief of dry, persistent, tickling coughs of dogs, for quieting and relaxing dogs, and for suppressing coughs.

Protection Against Quackery

Be Able to Recognize Quackery

Although governmental agencies are actively and fairly successfully combating quackery, there will always be some worthless treatments and products offered to the public. It takes time for the government to act, and a quack may escape government detection for a period of time.

It is therefore important for the individual to be able to recognize quackery and to know how to avoid it. Some of the signs of quackery are given below. Some of the signs discussed apply mainly to clinical quackery, where a "doctor" administers treatments or sells products directly to patients. Other signs apply more to the sale of nonprescription remedies through mail order, drugstores, and "health food" stores. Some of the signs apply to both forms of quackery.

Signs of Quackery
Boastful Advertising

The code of ethics of most medical, dental, and similar professional associations prohibits or greatly restricts the advertising of services by members. Generally, a simple announcement of name, address, and type of practice is all that is considered ethical. Large advertisements boasting of the ability to cure many kinds of diseases are seldom purchased by the ethical physician.

Offer of Free or Low-Cost Diagnosis

Less ethical practitioners often advertise complete physical examinations at very low costs ($10 or $15). The practitioner who gives a free or low-cost diagnosis must make a living from the treatments rendered, so he or she is naturally inclined to make a diagnosis which is going to lead to some of these treatments. These practitioners often treat perfectly healthy persons, or fail to detect serious disorders which a person may have.

Location

The ethical practitioner usually prefers a professional environment for an office. Medical offices, for example, are often near a hospital. The practitioner who rents space in a department store or discount store is not necessarily unethical, but one should be alert for other signs of quackery.

Claim to Cure Diseases That Others Cannot Cure

The quack often claims that he or she has the ability to cure some condition that the ethical physician cannot always cure, such as cancer, arthritis, or old age.

Guarantee of Cure or Satisfaction

The ethical physician never guarantees a cure; such a physician does the best he or she can, but medical science has not progressed to the point that results are that certain. Even with a personal guarantee, the quack is seldom known to refund any money.

Claims of Secret Treatments

Claims of secret machines and formulas are meaningless because the ethical physician has knowledge of all the latest treatments and has access to their use. The secret remedies of quacks, upon investigation, always turn out to be worthless.

Testimonial Letters

Quacks often make use of letters of testimonial; ethical practitioners seldom or never use this technique. No importance can be placed on these letters; many of them have been bought or are written by ignorant people who really never had any disease. Some testimonials are written by people who later died of the disease from which they claimed to have been cured.

Attacks against the Medical Profession

The quack often loudly attacks the medical profession for its extensive use of surgery and drugs. These are, of course, the most valuable treatments for many disorders; but the quack cannot legally use drugs or surgery so claims the superiority of his or her own methods of treatment.

The quack is often very defensive and claims that he or she is being persecuted by the medical associations and the government. Any practitioner who makes this claim should be regarded as a possible quack since it indicates that such a person uses unproven methods and has probably been in legal trouble as a result.

Diagnosis by Mail

Many mail-order advertisements invite you to mail in a description of your symptoms from which the proper medication is prescribed and mailed to you. This is *quackery*. Not even the most skilled physician could make an accurate diagnosis by mail.

Public Protection

Government Agencies

At every level of government, efforts are being made to control fraudulent health practices. The Federal Trade Commission is active in cases involving fraudulent or deceptive advertising. The Postal Service may move rapidly in cases of mail-order fraud. The Food and Drug Administration regulates the purity, safety, and proper labeling of drugs and food products moved across state lines. Certain state, county, and city governments are also active in suppressing quackery. In 1967 the state of California became a leader in the fight against quackery by enacting laws making fraudulent practices a felony.

Nongovernment Organizations

Several privately financed groups actively participate in the restraint of health frauds. Among these are the Bureau of Investigation of the American Medical Association, the Better Business Bureau, and the Chamber of Commerce. Although these organizations have no legal regulatory powers, they can bring cases of fraud to the attention of the public and the proper legal regulatory authorities.

When a person is in doubt about the merits of a particular product or treatment, it is often worthwhile to check with a local Chamber of Commerce, Better Business Bureau, local medical society, or a licensed and registered physician.

Persistence of Quackery

How does quackery persist in spite of intensive efforts by government and individuals to suppress it? The answer is that, although the quack might not be very skilled in treating disease, he is very adept in other areas. He often operates at the very borderline of legality, perhaps obeying the letter but not the spirit of the law. When convicted, he usually serves a short jail sentence and pays a stiff fine (which he can well afford); then, immediately, he changes his location and perhaps his name and is back in business again.

Often, even getting a conviction proves to be very difficult. Juries may be swayed by the emotional testimonies of former patients of the quack. Large corporations engaged in sales of proprietary compounds retain excellent lawyers to fight their battles with the authorities, and the corporations often win. For example, it took the federal government sixteen years to get the word "liver" removed from the name of Carter's Little (Liver) Pills on the basis that the pills had nothing to do with the liver.

The private citizen can aid in the campaign against quackery through reporting incidents of suspected quackery to the local district attorney's office or the local medical society. It is often only through such complaints that authorities are alerted to a fraudulent operation. It is apparent that today, as always, it is the responsibility of the individual to be alert to health fraud and quackery and to avoid them.

Summary

I. Who Are the Quacks?

  A. A few are licensed medical doctors

  B. Many have had limited training, as in chiropractic or naturopathic methods

  C. Some have had no training at all

  D. Self-treatment is quackery

II. Who Turns to Quackery?

    A. All kinds of people, especially the young and the elderly, the rich and the poor

    B. Fear, ignorance, and gullibility are the allies of the quack

III. Major Types of Quackery Today

    A. Cancer quackery

        1. Often delays effective treatment until the disease has become incurable

        2. Many people turn to quacks because of fear of surgery

    B. Arthritis quackery

        1. About half of all arthritics try quack remedies

        2. The ethical physician offers the best available treatments

    C. Food quackery

        1. Affects millions of Americans

        2. Products are often sold by scare tactics

            a. Myth that all disease is due to faulty diet

            b. Myth of the indispensable food product

            c. Myths about soil depletion

            d. Myths about "organic" or "natural" foods

            e. Myths about food processing

        3. Food quackery may result in malnutrition or delay in medical treatment for serious diseases

    D. "Reduce without dieting"

        1. There is no "easy" way to lose weight

        2. Schemes of little or no value include

            a. Nonprescription pills

            b. Spot reducing

            c. Vibrators

            d. Massaging devices

            e. Reducing creams

    E. Bust development

        1. Ineffective or dangerous schemes include

            a. Special exercises

  b. Special diets

  c. Breast development creams

  d. Silicone implants and injections

  2. The "flat" woman should realize that there is no relationship between breast size and sexual adequacy or femininity

IV. Some Specific Examples of Quackery

  A. Mail fraud cases reported by the Post Office Department

  1. Cancer cures

  2. Unneeded or worthless treatments

  3. Diet tablets

  4. Blessed handkerchiefs

  5. Male and female aphrodisiacs

  6. Products to restore lost youth

  B. Products seized by the Food and Drug Administration

V. Protection Against Quackery

  A. Be able to recognize the signs of quackery

  1. Boastful advertising

  2. Offers of free or low-cost diagnosis

  3. Unusual location

  4. Claims to cure diseases others cannot cure

  5. Guarantee of cure or satisfaction

  6. Claims of secret treatments

  7. Testimonial letters

  8. Attacks against the medical profession

  9. Diagnosis by mail

  B. Public protection

  1. Government agencies

  2. Nongovernmental organizations

  C. Persistence of quackery

  1. Borderline of legality

  2. Change of name and location

3. Emotional appeal of testimonies

4. All suspected quackery should be reported

Questions for Review

1. What are the basic forms of modern quackery?

2. What is a quack?

3. What formal training may a quack possess?

4. What groups of persons are especially susceptible to quackery?

5. Why may cancer quackery be particularly tragic?

6. What sales techniques are used in food quackery?

7. What are some possible dangers in food quackery?

8. Of the various bust-development plans, which offers the most hope without danger?

9. List some ways in which a quack may be detected.

10. Why does quackery still persist despite the intensive efforts of government agencies to suppress it?

Chapter 6
FINANCING HEALTH SERVICES

D eciding upon and/or obtaining quality health services is a primary concern of most adults. No less important is their being able to pay for such services. Today good health care is usually expensive.

Many people are perplexed about why good health care must cost as much as it does. Is it simply overpriced? Have the costs for all health services risen uniformly or are some rising faster than others? And if so, why? Although the average family is paying out more dollars for health care, is this care taking the same or a higher percentage of their take-home pay than it did in the past? Are people faced with scores of appealing consumer products giving as high a priority to quality health care as they should? Should it be the individual's responsibility to pay for all his or her health care, or should the government provide national health insurance as Canada now does?

In the midst of continuing public debate, the United States is moving toward a solution to the profoundly complex problems in the current system of health care and its financing. The basic concerns are the cost, distribution, and quality of health care services. The challenge is to bring to all the benefits of advanced medical technology and to achieve this end equitably, efficiently, and at reasonable cost.

Alternate approaches to the problem are being analyzed by the public and Congress. Essential to the issue is the role both the public and private sectors now play, and should play in the future, in the organization, delivery, and means of payment for health care.

Why the High Cost of Health Care?

Inflation has been a particular problem in the field of health care. The medical care portion of the Consumer Index (CPI) has risen faster than the average for all goods and services itemized in the CPI (Fig. 6.1). The American public spends an average of 59 percent more in health care now than 10 years ago. In terms of kinds of care, the total percentage increase breaks down this way: hospital care, up 166 percent; physicians' services, up 65 percent; dentists' services, up 56 percent; optometric examinations and eyeglasses, up 40 percent; and the cost of prescriptions and drugs, up 9 percent. For the same period of time, the amount spent for all personal items (including health care) increased only 38 percent.

Of the typical dollar spent for health care in the United States in 1972, 38 cents of the dollar was spent for hospital services, 28 cents for physicians' services, and 18 cents for medicines and appliances. Figure 6.2 shows how the entire dollar spent for health care was divided up.

There is no doubt that much of this higher cost represents proportionately better care. As previously mentioned, in a study from Massachusetts General Hospital, per patient cost for coronary care has increased from $200.00 per day in 1920 to $3500.00 per day in 1970. The benefit from such cost increases has been a drop in fatalities from 40 per 100 patients in 1920 to 16 per 100 patients in 1970.

In spite of past increases in medical costs, all indications are that if medical services are to be improved to any extent, the costs will go higher. Medical authorities predict that medical advances can be measured in terms of more expense, and that by the end of the 1970s, personal medical expenses will take no less than 8 percent of the gross national product. Already costs of 100 dollars per day per bed are common, with intensive care beds now averaging about 200 to 500 dollars per day.

Why the great increase in medical costs? Answers are multiple. Costs per square foot on new construction of hospitals have soared; hospital employee salaries and benefits are up (63 percent of the hospital budget goes into salaries and benefits); new equipment becomes obsolete before it is worn out. It is estimated that every year about half of the major equipment in a hospital becomes obsolete. Hospitals are expected to be open and available 24 hours a day, 365 days a year, emergency or not. A high-quality, acute-care hospital hires an average of six employees for every patient.

There is public apathy about hospital costs; people are confident that, unreasonable cost or not, their health insurance will bail them out (often

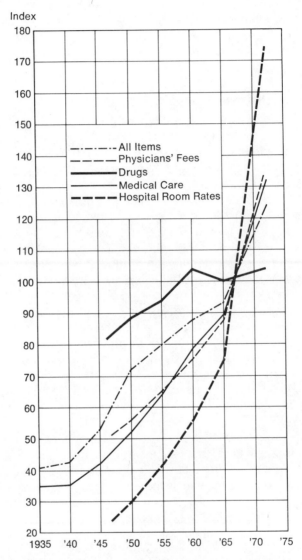

Figure 6.1. *Consumer Price Indices (CPI) for Medical Care Items in Comparison with the CPI for All Items in the United States (1967 = 100.0) (U.S. Department of Labor).*

unaware their insurance will pay only one-fourth to one-third of most hospital bills). Welfare payments are rarely enough to pay the true cost of public care. To make ends meet, hospitals overcharge private patients (and their insurance companies). Some private insurance policies provide coverage only if the patient is admitted to the hospital overnight (although overnight admission may not be required for the emergency). People abuse

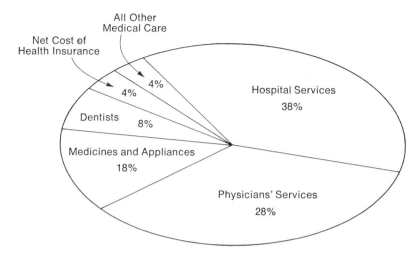

Figure 6.2. *Distribution of Personal Expenditures for Medical Care in the United States in 1972 (Health Insurance Institute, New York, N.Y., 1974).*

their health insurance—figuring the care is coming to them, they forget that each such unnecessary use helps boost the cost of health insurance. People go to the hospital when the same care might be provided just as well and with much less cost in a physician's office or clinic.

Although disturbing, there is evidence that the medical profession (at least the AMA) has been opposed to both better and cheaper medical care. Many physicians are guilty of greater concern over maintaining their high income than providing medical service their patients can afford. Medical care costs everyone. It should be used discreetly and only at those times it is required.

Paying Medical Bills

The traditional method of financing health costs has been for each family to pay off its medical bills as they arise, always hoping that there is sufficient money available in the bank to cover major episodes. For some families, this amounted to a "pay-as-you-go" method, hoping the money for the week would hold out; for others, it was a matter of budgeting, reserving money each month for medical costs. Were all medical expenses "average," it wouldn't be too difficult for a family to budget money each month for such a purpose, just like a budget for other household expenses. However, medical expenses are often erratic, with times of great expense separated by times of lesser expense, so that budgeting becomes almost impossible. All of us know of some families that seem to be hit repeatedly by heavy medical expenses which go far beyond the average. As a result of the erratic, unpredictable nature of medical costs for a family, there has been a greatly increasing trend toward collective financing of medical expenses.

It is the boast of the health insurance field that over 89 percent of our population holds some form of health insurance (Figure 6.3). Studies show that in the long run medical care tends to be a little cheaper in the form of a prepaid plan. In this manner people are protected somewhat against sudden large medical expenses by being forced systematically to lay away funds.

The current methods of collective financing of medical costs fall into one of two basic categories—public (tax-supported) and private (voluntary) health insurance.

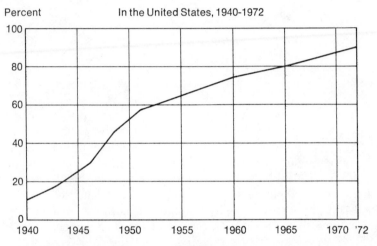

Figure 6.3. *Percentage of the U.S. population (consisting of civilian residents) with some form of health insurance protection, 1940–1972 (Health Insurance Institute; U.S. Department of Commerce, 1974).*

Public Medical Care

Care of the Poor

Most of the first organized medical programs were those for the poor. In the mid-1930s Congress passed the Federal Social Security Act. Among other things, this act provided medical services for several categories of poor people: the elderly, the blind, and dependent children. In January 1966 *Medicaid* (Title 19 of the Social Security Act) gave funds to states to expand their public assistance programs to persons, regardless of age, whose incomes are insufficient to pay for health care. *Medicaid* greatly increased medical care for the poor.

According to the Bureau of the Census, over 13.7 percent of all Americans live *below* the poverty line. By federal definition, the "poor are those who are not now maintaining a decent standard of living—those whose basic needs exceed their means to satisfy them."

While 68 percent of the poor are white, 32 percent are nonwhite. But the number of whites in our population greatly outnumber the nonwhites. A more accurate picture of poverty on a racial basis would be the ratio of white poor to all whites, and nonwhite poor to all nonwhites. Over 9 percent of *all* whites are poor, but over 32 percent of *all* nonwhites are poor.

One of the basic needs of people is adequate medical care. Those poor living in urban areas generally have greater access to such services than rural poor. Significantly, slightly over one-half of all poor families live in metropolitan areas, and slightly less than one-half in nonmetropolitan areas. Of all poor families in the country, almost one-half live in the South.

Although there are adequate health services available in most urban areas, gaps still exist in services provided for the rural poor. Shortages in hospitals, clinics, and physicians, and problems of patients having ready transportation for such services, still exist. The level of welfare payments for those unable to pay varies among the states. Southern states tend to provide less in public health care than any other region of the U.S.

Medicare

Medicare, a government program of health insurance under Social Security which helps the elderly (those sixty-five years of age and older) pay for medical care, became effective July 1, 1966. It has two parts: compulsory hospitalization financed by contributions from employees and employers, and voluntary medical insurance.

Hospital Insurance

The hospital insurance portion of Medicare helps pay for medical care received as a hospital in-patient and for certain follow-up services. It does not pay physicians' bills. Its basic coverage includes: (1) up to 90 days of in-patient care in any participating hospital in each benefit period (a new benefit period begins after a person has not been an in-patient for 60 days); (2) a "lifetime reserve" of 60 additional hospital days; (3) up to 100 days of care in each benefit period in a participating extended-care facility, such as a nursing home, after the patient leaves the hospital; and (4) up to 100 medically necessary home-health "visits" by nurses, physical therapists, home-health aides, or other health workers.

Medical Insurance

The medical insurance part of Medicare helps pay physicians' bills, as well as a number of other medical items and services not covered under hospital insurance. The plan is voluntary and people must sign up for it. Those who are drawing benefits before age 65 are enrolled in the medical insurance automatically. The monthly premiums, or payments, are shared equally by those who sign and by the federal government. A person can sign up for the medical insurance at age sixty-five whether or not he or she is eligible for other services of Medicare under Social Security.

Medical insurance benefits include payment for (1) physicians' services; (2) up to 100 home-health visits each year furnished by a home-health agency taking part in Medicare, if a physician arranges the treatment; (3) other medical health services prescribed by a physician, such as x-ray, radiation, artificial limbs, surgical dressings; and (4) office medical supplies, out-patient physical therapy services, and ambulance services.

A subscriber pays the first $60 of his or her medical expenses each year and 20 percent of the balance. A person can drop out of medical insurance at any time by filing written notice.

Military Coverage

A military veteran may receive care for any condition inflicted or activated during service. The veteran will be taken care of at government expense through the Veterans' Administration hospitals. Wives and children of military personnel who are on active duty or who are retired from the service are eligible for the Aid to Military Dependents Program. Children are covered until they are 18 years of age.

Special Groups

Medical care is provided for several unique groups for whom the federal government assumes responsibility. These are (1) *military personnel,* people on active military duty, (2) *United States Merchant Marines,* and (3) *American Indians,* through Public Health Service hospitals and clinics on the reservations.

Special Diseases

There are tax-supported medical programs for certain noncommunicable diseases that are of particular social concern. State hospitals for the mentally ill and neurologically disabled have been provided for almost 100 years. Clinics and hospitals for drug problems are on the increase both by the federal government and within the individual states.

Communicable Diseases

Communicable diseases are of high public concern. Venereal diseases (syphilis and gonorrhea) have reached epidemic proportions in this country. Public medical care centers, often city or county, provide public education, diagnosis, and treatment. There is a public hospital for lepers at Carville, Louisiana. In some of the larger cities there are special hospitals for other infectious diseases.

Crippled Children and Adults

Medical care for crippled children is usually administered by state health departments. Such children are eligible to receive both medical and educational services. Crippled children's programs generally have high medical standards and commonly require the services of medical specialists.

There are two basic kinds of organized medical-care programs for crippled adults. Workmen's Compensation Insurance is the older of these. Workmen's Compensation is not actually a tax-supported medical program in the sense that taxpayers pay for it directly. Rather, it is a form of insurance an employer is required by state law to carry for employees. It can be considered a public program in the sense that it is provided as the result of legislation. Workmen's Compensation insures the medical care of employees who are involved in industrial accidents. The second kind of program for crippled adults includes certain crippling conditions which may or may not be related to their employment, such as amputation, blindness, or crippling arthritis. Federal and state agencies sometimes cooperate on such programs because the patient is eligible not only for medical care but also for vocational retraining.

General Hospital Care

Most counties and larger cities in the country provide a county or general hospital for their citizens. Although these hospitals, such as the local community hospital, usually provide general medical care, they tend to be strongly oriented to the care of poor persons or those with chronic illnesses.

Local or County Health Departments

Virtually every county government in the United States supports some kind of county health department. Services provided vary from county to county, but usually include some or all of the following: (1) communicable disease control, (2) tuberculosis control, (3) venereal disease control, (4) local community health offices, (5) public health nursing service, (6) public health social services, (7) public health nutrition services (8) child and maternal health consultations, (9) public health dentistry, (10) sanitation inspection and supervision, (11) maintenance of vital records (births and deaths), (12) public health education, (13) air pollution control, and (14) school- and industrial-health services.

Eligibility for services from county health departments and general hospitals will vary from place to place and will depend upon the restrictions thought necessary by the local agency.

Private Health Insurance Programs

Over 89 percent of the total population within the United States is covered to some extent by some form of private health insurance (Figure 6.4).

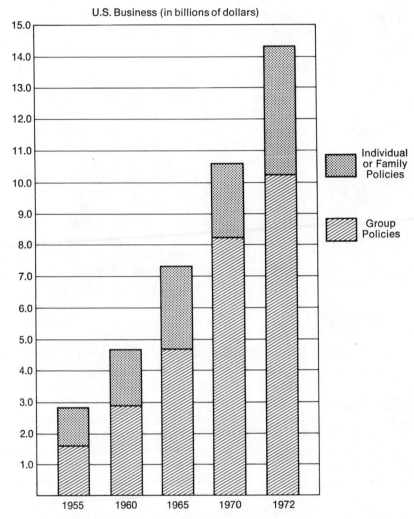

Figure 6.4. *Ratio of health insurance premiums of insurance companies by type of policy (Health Insurance Institute: New York, N.Y.).*

The whole reason for the existence of private health insurance programs is that individuals cannot successfully budget against the potential costs of all illnesses. This is surely true with certain illnesses, such as cancer, that may require long hospitalization and much medical care and could easily bankrupt the average family. The best hope for protection against these larger medical expenses, then, lies in large numbers of persons pooling the risks through insured health plans in which an insurance company agrees to provide certain health services for individuals. In return each policyholder pays a certain number of dollars to the insurance company monthly, quarterly, semiannually, or annually.

Unlike the public insurance plans, the costs of private health coverage are maintained solely by the beneficiaries. The major advantage of private health insurance at the present time is that it does permit the insured to select specific provisions and types of coverage that might be unavailable through public plans. Another advantage of private health insurance coverage is that it encourages the insured to take better care of themselves —to see a physician or have necessary diagnostic work done, knowing that they are already allotted a specific amount of money for this purpose. With Medicare in effect, most health care policies now terminate at age 65, or when the insured individual becomes eligible for Medicare.

Many insurance companies now sell medical insurance (also known as hospital or surgical insurance) through employee groups, professional organizations, and directly to individuals.

Kinds of Subscriptions

The most favorable premium rates (the cost of the insurance) have been gained through the formation of groups of subscribers (those who buy the insurance). A group is composed of a number of individuals or families who subscribe to a similar insurance plan. Group plans are generally available only through an employer. Typically, only one type of plan is available, with a similar premium charge to each subscriber within the group who holds a similar insurance contract (there may be some small differences in premium rate depending upon the size of the family). It generally costs more for an individual to buy insurance of the same type and coverage, or else the policy may contain fewer benefits. The majority of people covered by health insurance today belong to group plans (Figure 6.4). Group policies paid out in 1972 almost six times as many dollars in benefits as did the individual/family policies.

Types of Benefits

In terms of benefits (the services on which the insurance plan makes payment), there are two general types of plans: *service* and *cash indemnity* plans.

Service plans are generally in the form of contracts between the policyholder and the hospital or physician. The hospital agrees to provide certain services to anyone who is a policyholder under such a plan and who can present a policy identification card. The hospital or physician then agrees to accept the fees allowed under the plan as full or near-full payment for the care that is given. After the hospital (or physician) has completed its service, its office fills out a claim form and sends it to the insurance company. Reimbursement (payment) is then made directly to the hospital or physician according to the provisions of the policy.

Cash indemnity plans pay benefits in the form of cash to the policyholder, whereby the insured person is paid a specified sum of money toward covered expenses. (These payments can also be made directly to the provider of care through an arrangement called an assignment of benefits.) The patient is generally required to present either a physician's or hospital's statement showing the exact amount due or a receipt confirming payment already made.

Types of Insurers

There are no two health insurance plans that are exactly alike. There are several hundred different health insurance companies in the country today. Their plans, however, tend to fall into several main categories.

Blue Cross

Blue Cross is a nonprofit operation with over 68 million members. This represents about 38 percent of the population (one out of every three persons), and 84 percent of all Blue Cross members belong to a group plan. Through eighty plans in the United States, Blue Cross insures members against costs of hospital care, physicians' services, drugs, and laboratory tests. Even though all plans bear the name Blue Cross, each is sold exclusively within a given geographical area, and each is governed independently by a local board of community, hospital, and medical leaders who serve without compensation. Blue Cross is officially endorsed by the American Hospital Association.

Due to the diversity of Blue Cross plans across the country, no plan can be accurately described as typical. Each plan is serviced by a separate, regional, autonomous organization under the national name of Blue Cross. Each plan, therefore, sets its own policies, rates, and benefits, and makes its own contracts with hospitals in its territory. Each Blue Cross organization has the right to contract only with those hospitals and physicians which meet its standards of acceptability. Consequently, not all hospitals are eligible to receive Blue Cross payments. Subscribers receive benefits anywhere in the country. They can transfer from one Plan area to another and may adjust their coverage as their marital/family status changes.

Types of coverage range from several weeks to a full year of hospital service. The most widely sold policies cover the partial or complete cost of thirty days of hospital care. Other plans also cover services of physicians, anesthetists, x-ray diagnosis and therapy, drugs, and laboratory tests. Most plans also now include extended coverage (benefits payable in the event of a long siege of illness). Hospital claims are paid directly to the contracting hospital. Physician claims may be mailed to the subscriber (who endorses the check and mails it to the physician) or directly to the physician.

Blue Shield

Set up along the same general lines as Blue Cross, Blue Shield plans claim over 83 million subscribers through seventy-one different plans. Organized in 1946 and endorsed by the American Hospital Association, Blue Shield offers plans designed to provide prepaid coverage for physicians' services and at the same time help to assure the collection of physicians' fees. Payments of claims are made to physicians based either on their usual, customary, and reasonable (UCR) fee for the area, or on a fixed dollar amount for a given type of care. In some areas, such as Southern California, Blue Shield prepays both physician and hospital costs. Blue Shield is available in most states.

Commercial

Most of the health insurance plans available are written by commercial insurance companies (Figure 6.5). Although their coverage is similar to that of Blue Cross and Blue Shield, the approach of the commercial companies is often different. Their plans tend to be of the cash indemnity type or are a combination of service-cash indemnity. The commercial health insurance companies in no way engage in setting up contracts

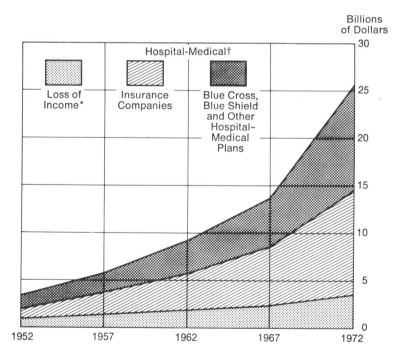

*Insurance companies only.

†Includes surgical, dental, and major medical premiums.

Figure 6.5. *Distribution of Health Insurance Premiums by Type of Insurer, 1952– 1972* (Source Book of Health Insurance Data, 1973–1974, *Health Insurance Institute, New York, N.Y.).*

with hospitals or physicians and thus do not seek to control the quality of medical services rendered to their policyholders. A wide variety of plans are available, even from one given company; thus, the policy for a given person or family can be tailor-made to his needs or wishes.

Commercial companies have helped in the development of certain other forms of health insurance such as the following:

1. *Major Medical.*   Just as the name implies, these plans are set up to give large amounts of coverage for major expenses. They are not designed nor intended to pay for smaller medical expenses the insured individual can easily pay out of his own pocket or expenses which can be covered by the regular type of health insurance plan. Accordingly, major medical plans usually contain a deductible clause, excluding payments on medical expenses under $100 in some plans and up to $500 in others. The policyholder is expected to pay this amount himself. Some plans state that, in addition, the insured must bear the cost of 20 to 25 percent of the expenses above the deductible amounts, with the insurance company paying the other 75 to 80 percent.

2. *Comprehensive plans.*   Contracts of this type are designed to provide regular (basic) medical care *plus* major medical coverage. They are designed to combine the best features of the other types of policies. They can be purchased either on a group or individual basis. Some Blue Cross plans now offer comprehensive coverage.

3. *Income (Disability Income) Insurance.*   A person may not realize his need for income protection until his income ceases. Many people look upon accidents and serious illness as things that happen to "other people." This coverage may be in the form of short-term or long-term protection. (Short-term policies are those with a maximum benefit period up to 2 years; long-term plans have benefit periods greater than 2 years.)

Most income contracts are written on a scheduled basis. The insured elects to take such coverages as he or she believes will benefit him or her. The insured can tailor a contract to his or her particular needs and ability to pay. The total premium will be determined by the kinds and amounts of coverages the insured takes, his or her occupation, age, and sex. Accident coverage may include: total disability, partial disability, loss of life, limb, or sight, and blanket medical expense. Sickness coverage may include: total disability, hospital room and board, surgical operation, in-hospital physician, and nurse expense.

The most important part of the contract is the provision for total or partial disability. Most companies use a 30-, 60-, or 90-day clause requiring that disability commence within this time period following the accident.

It is important that a person look carefully at the insuring clause in accident policies, since they are not uniform. Some refer to injury, while others refer to "accidental means" or "accidental bodily injury." Sickness policies may make no distinction between "his occupation" and "any occupation" as found in most accident contracts, and most are limited to a maximum payment period of 52 or 104 weeks.

Partial disability payments are usually available in accident policies either automatically or for an additional premium. Benefits may be 40 to 50 percent of total disability benefits, payable only if the insured is able to go to work.

Income benefits for sicknesses are not sold separately from accident income protection. It is likely that both will be issued in the same contract; a separate contract covering accidents usually is drawn up only for those who specifically request such a policy.

Independents

There are several hundred smaller local plans which have not yet been described. They have been organized by labor unions, corporate managements, physicians, and laymen. They tend to be unique in that most of them provide their own salaried physicians, their own clinics, and some, their own hospitals. They go under such names as Health Insurance Plan of Greater New York, Kaiser Foundation Health Plan, and the Community Health Association of Detroit. Patients are expected to use the staff physician who is provided and not to bring a nonstaff physician into the clinic or hospital. Plans lacking their own hospitals have agreements with other hospitals. Although the independents are generally local, this doesn't mean they are small. Many are large organizations. New York State and California have a number of such plans.

Dental Plans

Health plans are now available which provide coverage for specific items such as dentistry, drugs, and contact lenses. Dental care, as an example, has usually been excluded from health care plans except as necessary in cases of accident. Increasingly popular dental insurance usually provides coverage for oral examinations (including x-rays and cleaning), fillings, extractions, inlays, bridgework, and dentures, as well as oral surgery, root canal therapy, and orthodontics.

Dental plans are commonly set up as group plans. One leader in this field has been Group Health Dental Insurance, Inc., in New York State. Rates depend upon the type of coverage provided and the makeup of the particular group. Most coverage provides a limited amount of care, with the patient paying the balance of the cost. Usually excluded are dental services not considered necessary for normal chewing. Further information describing available dental care plans can be obtained by checking the Digest of Prepaid Dental Care Plans, U.S. Public Health Service, Washington, D.C.

Private Health Insurance Benefits

The bulk of health insurance benefits paid out to persons under 65 years of age goes toward the payment of hospital expenses. Figure 6.6 shows the full distribution of benefit payments by private health insurance companies.

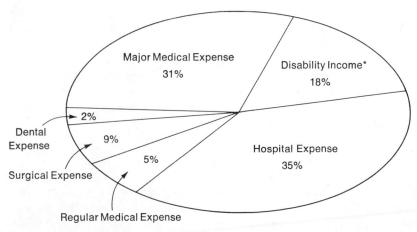

*Excludes accidental death and dismemberment benefits.

Figure 6.6. *Distribution of Health Insurance Benefit Payments Made by Insurance Companies by Type of Coverage, Under Age 65, for 1972 (Health Insurance Institute, New York, N.Y., 1974).*

Purchasing Health Insurance

The novice can easily be totally confused by first attempts at purchasing health, hospital, surgical, or accident insurance. Insurance can be literally a concern of life and death and should not become a battle of wits between the buyer and seller. Without too much trouble, the buyer can end up with a policy that does not provide the sort of coverage needed or provides essential coverage with a number of nonessential features included.

What to Look for When Purchasing Health Insurance

Overall, a person should determine: (1) the type of health care expenses he or she desires to be protected against and (2) the extent (proportion) to which he or she wishes these expenses insured.

Types of Health Care Expenses

There are three types of health care expenses: *hospital expenses, professional services* (performed by physicians licensed to practice medicine), and *paramedical services* (such as laboratory, x-ray, nursing, physical therapy, and pharmaceuticals). The first two types of expenses are more predictable and thus lend themselves more readily to the principles of insurance.

Extent of Coverage

A purchaser should consider the extent or proportion of the medical expenses he or she wants to have insured. The purchaser should have some idea what health-care expenses can amount to. It is wise to determine: (1) the prevailing hospitalization costs in your community, (2) the kinds of hospital services you prefer (private, semi-private, or ward), and (3) professional costs (information on prevailing physicians' charges in your community can be obtained from the physician or from a local medical-society office).

Underwriting Organization (the Insuring Company)

Here are some questions which should be answered about the insuring company.

1. Is the company or prepayment plan licensed to do business in your state?

2. What is the organization's reputation for fulfilling its obligations to its policyholders?

3. Is there a claims payment office located either in your state or otherwise reasonably near?

4. Does the company's agent have a good reputation in your community?

Contract Provisions

Contracts involve both privileges (benefits) and obligations. It is your absolute responsibility to read the contract and understand it *before* signing it (in spite of any insistence by the agent to do otherwise). Particularly, look for the following items.

1. *Insuring clause.* Be sure the coverage includes the types of benefits you desire.

2. *Exclusions or conditions not covered.* Most policies exclude certain benefits (the cost of the premium will be determined largely by the number and nature of the exclusions). Insurance companies commonly exclude the following: (1) plastic or cosmetic surgery; (2) elective surgery (that which can be done at the patient's convenience); some policies include such surgery six months or later from the date of purchase of the policy; (3) occupational illnesses and accidents covered by Workmen's Compensation; (4) conditions resulting from acts of war or riot (including injuries and illnesses sustained in the Armed Forces); (5) pre-existing illnesses; and (6) dental work.

3. *Waiting periods.* There is usually a time interval between the issuing of a contract and the date certain benefits are payable. Examples of such benefits might be maternity, elective surgery, or pre-existing illness. This provision is included because an insurance company usually agrees to cover only those conditions that commence after the insurance is written.

4. *Benefit reductions.* Benefits may be reduced below the amount otherwise payable. This may be done if the hospital is a noncontracting hospital with this company or if the physician is a nonparticipant.

5. *Persons covered.*   Usually the policy includes the spouse and unmarried dependent children; *these names must be specified in the policy.*

6. *Age limits.*   Some policies specify minimum and maximum age limits. Most policies will cover a dependent child only up to a stated age.

7. *Cancellation and renewal provisions.*   Many policies are cancelable by the insuring company; some policies state that the company can elect not to renew the policy at any premium-due date; some policies are both noncancelable and guaranteed renewable to a specified age (these may be more expensive but can be a better type of insurance).

8. *Limited choice of a physician or hospital.*   All limits should be explicitly understood. You should clearly understand whether your insurance is good if you are unable to use a designated hospital or physician —such as during travel or away-from-home employment.

Determining How Much Insurance You Can Afford

A person should have a clear picture of the regular, periodic payments he or she is obligated to pay—such as auto loan, rent or loan payment on a house, furniture payments, and auto insurance. A family must be sure that the expected health insurance premiums can be added to the budget and be paid. It is also wise to remember that the family with more financial obligations has as many, if not more, health insurance needs as the family with fewer financial obligations. If a financially obligated person were to encounter huge unexpected medical bills and not be able to keep up payments on his or her car, refrigerator, or house, these could be taken away through repossession or foreclosure. The financially obligated person *particularly* needs adequate health insurance. It must not be something a person plans to buy when all the rest of the bills have been paid.

Observing these points should enable a person to make a wise selection of health insurance. In certain types of employment the health insurance is automatically provided as a fringe benefit, and the employee does not need to select one policy as against another one. Further questions should be addressed to a person's insurance counselor, union office, or local Blue Cross or Blue Shield representative.

Clarification of Terms in Policy

In buying health insurance, or any other type of insurance, the purchaser should go over the policy word by word. He or she will also need to rely upon the reputation of the individual agent and the company issuing the policy.

If there are any questions pertaining to the wording of the policy, write out all the terms that are not completely clear, mail this to the main office of the insuring company and request a *letter of clarification*. Upon receiving such a clarification, study it carefully, then—and only then—sign the contract. Then clip the letter of clarification onto the policy. The insurance company is legally bound to the definitions contained within its policy and any letters of clarification.

Advice From a Physician or Hospital

Physicians and hospitals gain considerable experience in dealing with health insurance companies and usually have good ideas about which ones pay the benefits they claim to pay. If a person is in doubt as to which insurance company to select and which policy to choose, physicians and hospitals can generally give some rather accurate counsel. Hospitals will also be able to tell a person whether the benefits payable for specific hospital care are sufficient to pay for at least 80 percent of the hospital's charges:

Periodic Review of a Prepayment Plan

Every several years, it is a wise idea to take out your health insurance policy and read it. Be certain it still contains adequate coverage. While checking it, keep the following points in mind:

1. Changes may occur in a person's income, the relative needs of his or her family, and possibly the number in the family.

2. Employment may have changed. Some policies are carried with the employer, and a job layoff may cancel the policy.

3. There may have been a change of residence. Some policies are issued within a given geographical area and may not be in force in another area.

4. There may be changes in family situations—divorce, death, or birth. A man may still be carrying insurance for a divorced wife, whom he would prefer not insuring.

5. Check any other types of coverage you might be eligible for from other sources—Workmen's Compensation, sick leave, disability benefits, or any other health insurance. Normally, one company will not pay benefits for any claim that is covered by another insuring company.

Regardless of *how* a family provides for its medical care, there is no question that such care must be provided. Since most people must work and earn money, it is important that they protect themselves against the unexpected loss of income (since this loss could mean severe hardship for the family). A family must protect not only its ability to earn money, but also its savings and investments against large unanticipated medical and hospital costs. A well-planned, well-balanced health insurance program will do just this.

Summary

I. Why the High Cost of Medical Care?

   A. Hospital costs have risen 166 percent in the last ten years

B. However, percentage of a family's income spent on health care has risen only 59 percent in the same period.

II. Paying Medical Bills

A. ''Pay-as-you-go''

B. Collective financing through health insurance

1. Public—tax supported

2. Private—voluntary

III. Public Medical Care (Tax-Supported)

A. Care of the poor (indigent)—largely through Social Security and Medicare

B. Medicare—primarily for those over sixty-five years of age

1. Hospital insurance—helps pay portion of medical care received as hospital in-patient and for certain follow-up services

2. Medical insurance—helps pay portion of physicians' bills and certain other medical items and services

C. Military coverage—for veterans and families of military personnel

D. Special groups—military personnel, Merchant Marine, American Indians

E. Special diseases—most states provide hospitals for the emotionally and neurologically disabled and some, for drug problems

F. Communicable diseases—venereal diseases, leprosy

G. Crippled children and adults

H. General hospital care—most counties and larger cities in country provide county or general hospitals for residents

I. Local or county health departments

1. Provided by virtually every county in country

2. Services vary but may be quite extensive

IV. Private Health Insurance Programs

A. Over 89 percent of all United States population covered with some form of private health insurance

B. Kinds of subscriptions

1. Individual or family

2. Group (usually through employer)

C. Types of benefits

1. Service plans—contract between policyholder and hospital or physician

2. Cash indemnity plans—benefits in form of cash from insurance company directly to policyholder

D. Types of insurers

    1. Blue Cross

        a. Nonprofit plans providing hospital care, physicians' services, drugs, and laboratory tests

        b. Eighty different plans

    2. Blue Shield

        a. Follows same general lines as Blue Cross

        b. Through seventy-one different plans, primarily covers physicians' services

    3. Commercial

        a. Plans tend to be of cash indemnity type

        b. Highly variable; widely sold

        c. Have spearheaded

            (1) Major medical plans—give large coverage for major expenses

            (2) Comprehensive plans—provide basic medical care plus major medical coverage

            (3) Income (disability) plans—give income protection during disability from accident and/or sickness

    4. Independents

        a. Provide clinics, salaried physicians, and, in some cases, hospitals

        b. Kaiser Foundation Health Plan, Health Insurance Plan of Greater New York, Community Health Association of Detroit

    5. Dental Plans

V. Purchasing Health Insurance

    A. What to look for when purchasing health insurance

        1. Types of health care expenses that need to be covered

        2. Extent of coverage desired

        3. Underwriting organization (the insuring company)

        4. Contract provisions

            a. Insuring clause—scope of coverage

            b. Exclusions or conditions not covered in policy

            c. Waiting periods—before certain benefits are payable

            d. Benefit reductions

            e. Persons covered

      f. Age limits

      g. Cancellation and renewal provisions

      h. Limited choice of physician or hospital

   B. Determining how much insurance you can afford

      1. Must be enough to cover certain obligations that must be met

      2. Family must be able to meet premiums

   C. Clarification of terms in policy

      1. Questions regarding policy should be cleared up with letter to company home office

      2. Letter of clarification should be retained

   D. Advice from a physician or hospital

      1. Very useful in telling which company to choose

      2. Can counsel you on needed coverage

VI. Periodic Review of a Prepayment Plan

   A. Changes in a person's income or family

   B. Change in employment

   C. Change in residence

   D. Changes in family situations

   E. Be sure you know what other forms of coverage you might already have through other policies

Questions for Review

1. During the past decade health care costs have increased faster than the Consumer Price Index. What parts of medical costs have increased fastest and for what reasons?

2. In what ways has the "pay-as-you-go" method of financing health care been inadequate?

3. Distinguish between the two current methods of collective financing of health costs.

4. What are some of the groups of people who have received tax-supported health care?

5. In order to obtain the most favorable private health insurance, what should a person look for in terms of kinds of subscription, type of benefit, and type of insurer?

6. Describe Blue Cross in terms of type of coverage, how claims are paid, who its subscribers are, and for what each plan is responsible.

7. Compare major health insurance with comprehensive insurance.

8. What are some advantages in subscribing to an independent health insurance plan rather than to Blue Cross?

9. What two basic questions should a person answer before purchasing health insurance?

10. An underwriting (insuring) company should be considered by a potential client only if it can satisfy what four questions?

11. List and explain eight contract provisions which are commonly written into health insurance policies.

12. Give three types of health care expenses commonly covered in insurance plans.

13. On what point can a person determine how much insurance he or she can afford?

14. What is a letter of clarification and what is its importance?

15. A periodic review of one's health insurance policy should check what points?.

16. In what way might a physician or hospital be of assistance in determining subscription into a health insurance company?

HEALTH CAREER FIELDS

Today there are opportunities of many kinds in the health fields. Owing to the expanding and aging population in this country, rising awareness of health in the population, the explosion of health insurance plans, and the health care provisions under federal and state medical programs, the urgent need for many more health workers will continue. These professions cover all types of work and interests

Vocation	Nature of the Work	Education
Cytotechnologist	Does microscopic analysis of detached body cells to determine presence or absence of cancer, evaluates estrogen, stains slides.	At least 2 years of college work with emphasis on biology courses, followed by a 1 year clinical training program in an approved school of cytotechnology.
Dental Assistant	Prepares patients for examination or treatment, prepares dental materials, takes and processes x-rays, handles records, and serves as a receptionist.	Often training is given on the job. Some colleges are now giving a 1–2 year training program following high school graduation.

related to hospitals, clinics, laboratories, pharmacies, private offices, industrial plants, and nursing homes. They may require training lasting from a few months to many years and may be either routine or highly creative.

The following chart lists information regarding the various health careers. It has been designed to help a person decide if he or she belongs in one of these health fields.

Where Employed	Employment Opportunities	Where to Find Additional Information
Hospitals, clinics, or public health laboratories.	Increasing demand as cancer-diagnosing techniques improve. Some become laboratory supervisors.	Council of Medical Education, American Medical Assn., 535 N. Dearborn St., Chicago, Ill. 60610.
Dental offices and dental clinics.	Opportunities are easy to find. Advancements are limited.	American Dental Assistants Assn., 211 E. Chicago Ave., Chicago, Ill. 60611

Vocation	Nature of the Work	Education
Dental Hygienist	Cleans and polishes teeth, massages gums, charts conditions of decay and disease for diagnosis by a dentist, provides dental health education.	Usually a 2-to-4 year training program following high school leading to a dental hygiene certificate. A state board examination is required in most states, which, if passed, entitles one to become a Registered Dental Hygienist (R.D.H.).
Dental Laboratory Technician	Makes artificial dentures of all kinds upon prescription from a dentist. (Some do only selected kinds of work.) May work for one or several dentists and have no patient contact.	Commonly trained on the job—usually in a laboratory or dental school for 4–5 years. A few schools offer a 2-year training program.
Dentist	Fills cavities in the teeth, straightens teeth, x-rays the mouth, extracts teeth, substitutes artificial dentures, and treats gum diseases. Most dentists are in general practice. A few do research or teach either part-time or full-time.	Two to 3 years of college work followed by 4 years of dental training leading to the degree of Doctor of Dental Surgery (D.D.S.) or Doctor of Dental Medicine (D.M.D.). State board examinations required in most states. Advanced training required for dental specialties.
Dietician	Plans and supervises food preparations and meals, usually in hospitals, schools, or industry. Some are administrators, others are therapeutic dieticians, teachers, or research workers.	A bachelor's degree with a major in foods and nutrition or institution management. Often an internship program is required, as with medical therapeutic dietary work.

Where Employed	*Employment Opportunities*	*Where to Find Additional Information*
A profession consisting almost entirely of women, who work in private dental offices, public health agencies, industrial plants, or public school systems.	Future is increasingly good as dental care becomes more important. With a college degree, openings are good in public health.	Division of Educational Services, American Dental Hygienists' Association, 211 E. Chicago Ave., Chicago, Ill., 60611.
Commercial laboratories with 1–10 persons handling orders from many dentists. Some employed by private dentists, in hospitals, or by governmental agencies.	Job futures very good as dental care expands. Opportunities are good to set up one's own laboratory.	American Dental Assn., Council on Dental Education, 211 E. Chicago Ave., Chicago, Ill., 60611. National Association of Dental Laboratories, Inc., 3801 Mt. Vernon Ave., Alexandria, Va. 22305.
Mostly in private practice, others in armed services, dental schools, hospitals, and public health.	Demand for dentists is growing faster than the supply for private practice, public health, research, and dental college faculties.	American Dental Association, Council on Dental Education, 211 E. Chicago Ave., Chicago, Ill., 60611. American Association of Dental Schools, 1625 Massachusetts Ave., N.W., Washington, D.C. 20036.
Hospitals, school systems, colleges, industrial plants, public health departments, and private food service companies.	Need will continue to be high for a number of years as public health programs rapidly increase. Number of men in field is small but slowly increasing.	The American Dietetic Association, 620 N. Michigan Ave., Chicago, Ill., 60611.

Vocation	Nature of the Work	Education
Environmental Engineer or Technician	Detects, analyzes, and measures environmental hazards; determines effects of hazards; develops standards of pollution; and sets up programs to control or prevent hazards.	Bachelor's degree in some phase of engineering (engineer); bachelor's degree in environmental health or in physical or biological sciences (technician). Some graduate programs with master's or doctorate degrees.
Food Scientist (Food Technologist)	Concerned with all phases of production, processing, packaging, distribution and utilization of foods; checks food spoilage and quality control; may teach or give consultation.	Generally a bachelor's degree in food science or in chemistry or biology. Some schools offer graduate programs.
Hospital Administrator	In charge of the hospital management, its smooth running, and the carrying out of board policies. In charge of all departments, staff members, and facilities. Responsible for hiring, training, budgets, planning, purchasing, and accounting.	New people in the field have master's or Ph.D. degrees in hospital administration, law, or business administration. Some must be physicians or registered nurses. Internships required in some states.
Industrial Hygienist	Watches factory environment for anything of possible harm to employees and recommends necessary changes.	Bachelor's degree with major in physical sciences. Some go on for master's degree in public health.
Medical Assistant	Helps prepare patients for examinations, sterilizes instruments, records information, and runs routine tests. Works under a nurse or physician. If in a laboratory, probably works under a technologist or a pathologist.	Often expected to have some college training in biological sciences. Some junior colleges offer 2-year programs with special work in medical records, terminology, and laboratory procedures.

Where Employed	Employment Opportunities	Where to Find Additional Information
Federal, state, or local government; public health laboratories; private industry.	Relatively new fields. Limitless opportunities with urgent need for more workers. Openings as educators, inspectors, advisors.	American Public Health Association, 1015 18th St. N.W., Washington, D.C. 20036.
Canning factories and research departments of food industries and manufacturers.	Field rather new and a number of opportunities for work are open. The better the training, the better the job opportunities.	American Home Economics Association, 1600 20th St. N.W., Washington, D.C., 20009. The Institute of Food Technologists, Suite 2120, 221 N. LaSalle St., Chicago, Ill. 60601.
Hospitals of all kinds and related institutions, both private and governmental.	Jobs increasing as number of new hospitals increases. First jobs are often as assistants or in a small hospital, and then eventually to full administrators in a large hospital if work is acceptable.	American College of Hospital Administrators, 840 N. Lake Shore Dr., Chicago, Ill., 60611. Association of University Programs in Health Administration, One Dupont Circle N.W., Washington, D.C., 20036.
Governmental health agencies, industry, insurance companies, consultant companies, and universities.	Profession is uncrowded. Work is demanding and calls for a responsible person.	American Public Health Association, 1015 18th St. N.W., Washington, D.C., 20036.
Hospitals, clinics, and physicians' offices.	Always openings in private physicians' offices. Better chance for advancement in hospitals or laboratories as supervisors.	American Medical Assn. Council on Medical Education, 535 N. Dearborn St., Chicago, Ill., 60610. American Assn. of Medical Assistants, One East Wacker Dr., Suite 1510, Chicago, Ill. 60601.

Vocation	Nature of the Work	Education
Medical Laboratory Assistant	Performs routine laboratory work under supervision of medical technologists—performs tests, prepares tissue samples and slides, takes blood samples, keeps records of tests, cleans and sterilizes laboratory equipment.	Training in a special school, hospital, or junior college (two-year programs). Further training can prepare one for medical technology.
Medical Record Administrator (Librarian)	Keeps complete and accurate records of all patients while in the hospital, their x-ray reports, laboratory reports, progress notes, etc; checks, organizes, and files them; compiles statistics; and summarizes the medical records.	Preferred training is 2–4 years of college work plus a 1-year course in medical record library service. Some hospitals offer in-service training programs. Librarians who are graduates of approved schools may take a national registration examination, and, if they pass, become Registered Record Librarians (R.R.L.).
Medical Social Worker	Helps patients and families with personal problems resulting from illness or disability. Helps with new job placement, convalescence, and any other needs.	Bachelor's degree plus 2 years of graduate study in medical social work, leading to a master's degree.
Medical Technologist	Does laboratory procedures of all kinds under the guidance of a physician or a pathologist as a part of the diagnosis of diseases. Some work in laboratories; others do new drug research or administer laboratories.	New students should take 3 years of college work in the sciences, plus 1 year of specialized laboratory training. Graduates of AMA-approved schools may take an examination to qualify for certification by the Registry of Medical Technologists of the International Society of Clinical Laboratory Technologists. Some states license medical technologists.

Where Employed	*Employment Opportunities*	*Where to Find Additional Information*
Hospital laboratories, private clinics, physicians' offices, public health, and pharmaceutical laboratories.	Excellent through 1970's.	Board of Certified Laboratory Assistants, 445 N. Lake Shore Dr., Chicago, Ill., 60611.
Hospitals, clinics, public health agencies, medical departments of insurance agencies, and industrial firms.	Many hospitals lack trained record librarians. Field is quite short of enough trained librarians. Mostly women, but a small number of men in the field.	American Association of Medical Record Librarians, 211 E. Chicago Ave., Chicago, Ill., 60611.
Hospitals, clinics, public and private health centers and departments. Some in teaching.	Many more openings than available workers.	National Assn. of Social Workers (Medical Social Work Section), 2 Park Ave., New York, N.Y., 10017.
Hospitals, private physicians' offices, clinics, public health laboratories, private laboratories, and drug manufacturers.	Demand is great. Good chance for advancement as supervisor or researcher. Fits in well as a part-time job.	American Society of Medical Technologists, 555 West Loop South, Houston, Texas, 77025. Board of Registry of the American Society of Clinical Pathologists, Box 4872 Chicago, Ill. 60680.

Vocation	Nature of the Work	Education
Nursing Aide	Shares in the actual care of patients, such as answering calls, feeding and bathing, and adjusting beds. Male aides are called orderlies.	No formal preparation required. Hospitals provide on-the-job training. No licensing required.
Nurse, Licensed Practical (L.P.N.)	Also known as a Licensed Vocational Nurse (L.V.N.). Assists in care of the physically and mentally ill under direction of physicians and registered nurses. Duties may include taking temperatures, bathing, taking blood pressure readings, etc.	A 1-year training program and passing a state examination for licensing. Practical nurses having no formal training are not eligible for licensing, thus only formally trained practical nurses may become L.P.N.'s.
Nurse, Registered Professional (R.N.)	Provides nursing services for patients, either by direct care or through supervising allied nursing personnel. Administers drugs prescribed by a physician, observes and records patient information, assists in patient education and rehabilitation , instructs other personnel and students, or does administrative work.	Several programs may be followed: (1) a 2-year program with A.A. degree, (2) a 3-year program with diploma or A.A. degree, or (3) a 4-year program integrated with academic work for bachelor's degree. A nurse may be registered by passing a state board examination (R.N.).
Nutritionist	Teaches people about food needs and helps special groups with adequate diets. Determines how food is utilized and its contents. Sees that scientific knowledge on foods is translated into simple, specific information people can understand and use.	College work with a home economics major, with special emphasis on foods, nutrition, and related sciences and with some work in the social sciences. Many have a year or more of graduate training.

Where Employed	Employment Opportunities	Where to Find Additional Information
Hospitals, nursing homes, and clinics.	Duties and responsibilities depend on size of hospital. Demand is constant wherever there are hospitals. Often a good job for young men and women seeking part-time work.	ANA Committee on Nursing Careers, American Nurses' Assn., 2420 Pershing Rd., Kansas City, Mo., 64108.
Hospitals, public health agencies, private homes, physicians' offices, nursing homes, and similar institutions.	Great shortage. Future employment quite secure. Little chance for advancement except in specialized areas. A few men in field help provide care for men patients.	ANA Committee on Nursing Careers, American Nurses' Assn., 2420 Pershing Rd., Kansas City, Mo., 64108. National Federation of Licensed Practical Nurses, Inc., 250 W. 57th St., New York, N.Y., 10019.
Public and private hospitals, public health nursing, industrial nursing, nursing education, private duty, clinics, private physicians' offices.	Continuing excellent demand in all parts of the country. Work often begins as general duty nurse. Chances good for advancement to supervisory or administrative position.	ANA Committee on Nursing Careers, American Nurses' Assn., 2420 Pershing Rd., Kansas City, Mo., 64108.
In hospitals as dieticians, in teaching, or in extension work. Many work in local public nutrition programs as teachers or consultants. Also in research or in college or university teaching.	County extension departments, local health departments, food industries, or universities. Advancement depends on amount of training and experience.	American Home Economics Association, 2010 Massachusetts Ave. N.W., Washington, D.C., 20036.

Vocation	Nature of the Work	Education
Occupational Therapist	Works under a physician and uses creative, educational, and recreational activities to help people get well both physically and mentally and to acquire job skills. Recommends activities to patients in terms of their likes, dislikes, and abilities.	Four years of college training leading to B.S. degree in occupational therapy, or 18 months of training after a bachelor's degree in some other field. Training includes both academic and clinical phases. Passing of national registration examination entitles therapist to registration and use of initials O.T.R.
Operating Room Technician	Also known as surgical technician. Assists in the care of patients in the operating room and/or delivery room and in the care, preparation, and maintenance of sterile and nonsterile supplies and equipment.	No formal educational requirements. Persons receive in-service training in hospitals. A few programs for high school graduates in vocational or trade schools.
Optician, Dispensing	Interprets prescription of optometrist or ophthalmologist for the grinding and polishing of lenses. Advises on selection of frames and shapes of lenses in terms of the facial features. Fits and adjusts the finished glasses.	Most get informal on-the-job training. With an apprenticeship program of 3–4 years, he or she may become an optical dispenser. Several schools offer courses. About one-third of the states license the technician or the dispenser of eyeglasses.
Optometrist	Examines eyes and performs other services to safeguard and improve vision. Uses special instruments to find eye defects and measure them. Does not use drugs or do surgery.	Usually 2 years of college work followed by 4 years of optometry training leading to degree Doctor of Optometry (O.D.). Passing a state board examination is required in all states.

Where Employed	*Employment Opportunities*	*Where to Find Additional Information*
Primarily a field for women, although men are entering it. Works in hospitals, rehabilitation centers, nursing homes, outpatient clinics, and research centers.	Need for many more registered therapists is extensive. Opportunities to move into research, administration, and teaching.	American Occupational Therapy Association, 6000 Executive Blvd., Rockville, Md., 20852.
In hospitals.	Opportunities will continue to increase as hospitals use more technical personnel to help assist the overloaded physician.	Assn. of Operating Room Technicians, Inc., 1100 West Littleton Blvd., Suite 101, Littleton, Colo., 80120.
Wholesale or large retail establishments or as dispenser owning one's own business. Some in optical laboratories.	Need will continue to increase as population expands. Advancement opportunities for supervisors or shop foremen in large establishments.	Associated Opticians of America, 1250 Connecticut Ave., N.W., Washington, D.C., 20036.
Usually self-employed. May start as an associate with established practitioner, be salaried in an industrial plant, or work in governmental agency.	Employment opportunities are good, particularly in private practice.	American Optometric Association, 7000 Chippewa St., St. Louis, Missouri, 63119.

Vocation	Nature of the Work	Education
Orthotist, Prosthetist	*Orthotist* makes and fits braces and other supports; *prosthetist* makes artificial arms and legs and adjusts them to fit amputees.	Apprentice training in a certified establishment where appliances are fitted and made. A few 2-year programs leading to A.A. degree or 4-year programs leading to B.A. degree. Can apply for certification after 4 years of work.
Osteopathic Physician	Treats illness and disease, giving special attention to impairments of the musculo-skeletal system. Makes major use of manipulative therapy along with drugs and surgery; uses other methods of prevention, diagnosis, and treatment, depending upon the individual patient.	Three to 4 years of preosteo-pathic training, 4 years of professional training leading to degree Doctor of Osteopathy (D.O.) followed by 12 months internship in a hospital; 2–5 years additional training required for specialties followed by 2 years of supervised practice in the specialty. Passing of state board examination required for practice.
Pharmacist	Specializes in science of drugs. Understands composition and effects of drugs, tests for purity and strength, and compounds them. Makes drugs and medicines available and gives information on their use; provides other kinds of medical supplies.	At least 5 years of professional study beyond high school leading to degree of Bachelor of Science in Pharmacy, followed by 1 year of practical experience under the supervision of a registered pharmacist. Some take advanced work. State board examination required in all states for a license to practice.
Physical Therapist	Helps persons with muscle, nerve, joint, and bone diseases or injuries. Under a physician's direction, helps patients overcome their disabilities through exercise, manipulation, or use of mechanical apparatuses. Teaches patients and families to perform exercises. Helps patients learn to live with limitations.	A 4 year training program, with most programs leading to a bachelor's degree or the master's degree. License to practice required in most states after having passed a state board examination.

Where Employed	Employment Opportunities	Where to Find Additional Information
Retail establishments, hospital shops, rehabilitation centers, or in small shops working alone or supervising other employees.	Employment is steady. Skilled fitters are needed more now than before. Opportunity to set up own shop and supervise other employees.	American Orthotic and Prosthetic Association, 919 18th St. N.W., Washington, D.C., 20006.
Usually in private practice or in partnership in clinics.	Excellent, particularly in parts of the country where osteopathy is an accepted form of treatment. Advancement in terms of location and size of practice and degree of training.	American Osteopathic Association, 212 E. Ohio St., Chicago, Ill., 60611.
Many in retail pharmacies, either as owner or as salaried employee. Others in pharmaceutical manufacturing or wholesaling, in hospitals, research or teaching.	Great need for well trained pharmacists. Opportunities to acquire own business and supervise other employees as one gains experience.	American Pharmaceutical Association, 2215 Constitution Ave. N.W., Washington, D.C., 20037. American Council on Pharmaceutical Education, 77 W. Washington St., Chicago, Ill., 60602.
Hospitals, children's hospitals, nursing homes, rehabilitation centers, industrial clinics, schools for crippled children, armed forces, and public health services.	Rapidly growing field. Not nearly enough workers. Many advance to teaching, research, or supervision. Many therapists are women.	American Physical Therapy Association, 1156 15th St. N.W., Washington, D.C., 20036.

Vocation	Nature of the Work	Education
Physician	Diagnoses diseases and treats people who are ill or in poor health. Concerned with prevention of disease and rehabilitation of people who are injured or ill.	Three to 4 years of college work, 4 years of professional training leading to degree Doctor of Medicine (M.D.), followed by a 1-year hospital internship. Passing a state or national board examination required for a license to practice; 2–4 years more training required for specialties.
Podiatrist	Diagnoses and treats diseases and deformities of the feet. Performs foot surgery, uses drugs and therapy, prescribes proper shoes, fits corrective devices, and provides general foot care.	Two years of college followed by 4 years of professional training after which the degree Doctor of Podiatric Medicine (D.P.M.) is awarded. A few states require a 1-year internship. License to practice granted upon passing of state board examination.
Psychiatric Social Worker	Attends patients in mental hospitals or clinics, often works in clinical teams with other kinds of professional personnel. Guides patients and families in understanding an illness and making social adjustments in homes and communities.	Bachelor's degree with a major in social sciences and a master's degree from a school of social work, which includes both academic and clinical study.
Psychiatric Technician	Also known as a Mental Health Aide or Assistant, is in charge of patient care and supervision in the ward.	No formal educational requirements in all states. Some states now requiring a one year vocational training program beyond high school.
Psychologist	Studies the behavior of persons and groups, helps them to understand themselves and achieve a satisfactory personal adjustment.	Generally a master's degree in psychology and often a Ph.D. degree, plus 1 year of clinical internship for clinical or counseling psychology.

Where Employed	*Employment Opportunities*	*Where to Find Additional Information*
Usually engaged in private practice. Others in armed services, veterans' hospitals, public health, industry, medical schools, state and local health departments, research, or professional organizations.	Opportunities are innumerable. Heavy demand for physicians. Good chance for advancement in many areas. A small percentage are women.	Council on Medical Education, American Medical Association, 535 N. Dearborn St., Chicago, Ill., 60610. Association of American Medical Colleges, One Dupont Circle N.W., Washington, D.C., 20036.
Usually in private practice. May be in hospitals, teaching, veterans' hospitals, the armed services, or industry.	Field is not overcrowded. Demand is growing. Advancement depends on size of practice. A few are women.	American Podiatry Association, 20 Chevy Chase Circle, N.W., Washington, D.C., 20015.
Mental hospitals and mental health clinics, child guidance centers, general hospitals, courts, and rehabilitation centers.	Openings are numerous and and increasing. A few top administrative positions are open for those with sufficient experience.	National Assn. of Social Workers, 15th and H St. NW., 600 Southern Bldg., Washington, D.C. 20005.
In psychiatric hospitals.	Opportunities will continue to increase.	Division of Health Careers, American Hospital Association, 840 North Lake Shore Drive, Chicago, Ill., 60611.
Teaching, research, hospitals, public schools, counseling clinics, government agencies, and personnel work.	Good for well-trained persons. A few administrative positions for those with experience.	American Psychological Association, 1200 17th St. N.W., Washington, D.C., 20036.

Vocation	Nature of the Work	Education
Psychometrist	Specializes in administering tests under guidance of a psychologist and interpreting the scores.	Ordinarily a master's degree in psychology, including 1 year of supervised experience.
Public Health Administrator	Directs professional health services. Work will vary considerably with nature of the service, but may consist of medical services in health agency, public service department, medical laboratory, or nursing service. Often works under a director to carry out general assignments.	Often bachelor's degree or master's degree in public administration, public health, or social science. May hold degree in specialized health fields such as medicine, nursing, or medical technology.
Public Health Educator	Specializes in getting health facts accepted and used. Works closely with community and professional groups to achieve projects and actions that maintain and improve health of the community.	Bachelor's degree in the sciences and the communication arts. Master's degree in public health if possible. Older health educators are often from other health fields.
Radiologic Technologist	Also called Medical X-ray Technician; operates x-ray equipment under general direction of physician. May work in research center or medical laboratory. Prepares radioisotope materials, records their use, maintains safety precautions.	Usually a 2-year training program beyond high school or junior college in a hospital or medical school (a few schools offer 3–4 year programs with a bachelor's degree). Registration by the passing of an examination with the American Registry of Radiologic Technologists (ARRT) desirable.
Respiratory Therapist (Inhalation Therapist)	Aids physicians in administering medical gases and in resuscitation procedures. Checks hospital's supply of oxygen and the safety rules in its use.	Following high school graduation, a 9-month in-service training program or a 2- or 4-year college program.

Where Employed	*Employment Opportunities*	*Where to Find Additional Information*
Usually works in association with or under supervision of a psychologist in schools, clinics, hospitals, and industry.	Increasing need as more public schools administer placement tests. Kind of advancement depends upon the nature of the particular job.	American Psychological Association, 1200 17th St. N.W., Washington, D.C., 20036.
Health agencies of all kinds.	All health agencies are looking for good managerial personnel. Advancement possibilities are excellent with training and successful experience.	American Public Health Association, 1015 18th St. N.W., Washington, D.C., 20036.
Local, state, and federal health departments, international health programs, extension services, hospitals, clinics, and industry.	A relatively new field. Urgent need for more. Advancement chances are good for administration and consultantships.	American Public Health Association, 1015 18th St. N.W., Washington, D.C., 20036.
Hospitals, medical laboratories, clinics, physicians' and dentists' offices, school systems, or governmental agencies.	The shortage of technicians is expected to continue as more hospitals and medical facilities are built.	The American Society of Radiologic Technologists, 645 North Michigan Ave., Chicago, Ill., 60611. The American Registry of Radiologic Technologists, 2600 Wayzata Blvd., Minneapolls, Minn., 55405.
Hospitals, clinics, research laboratories, and offices.	Opportunity will depend on the size of the hospital and the kind of work called for.	American Association of Respiratory Therapy, 7411 Hines Place, Dallas, Tex. 75235.

Vocation	Nature of the Work	Education
Sanitarian (Environmentalist)	Determines standards and enforces regulations for food, milk, air, water, radiation, metropolitan planning, accident prevention, hospital sanitation, rodent control, housing, industrial hygiene, sewage and waste disposal.	Bachelor's degree in sciences, humanities, or communication arts. Master's degree in public health or related health field recommended.
Speech Pathologist and Audiologist	Identify and evaluate speech and hearing disorders using diagnostic procedures. Some do research work or teach in colleges or universities.	Bachelor's degree in speech, biological sciences, physics, and related areas in college or university; master's degree in speech pathology or audiology.

Where Employed	*Employment Opportunities*	*Where to Find Additional Information*
Local, state, and federal health departments, industry, hospitals, schools and colleges, federal agencies (Public Health Service), and international agencies (Peace Corps, World Health Organization).	Relatively new field. Limitless opportunities with urgent need for more workers. Openings in public health as educators, inspectors, and advisors.	National Environmental Health Assn., 1600 Pennsylvania St., Denver, Colo., 80203. American Public Health Association, 1015 18th St. N.W., Washington, D.C., 20036.
Public school systems and clinics, colleges and universities, hospitals, research centers, and private practice.	Good through 1970s, particularly for those who have completed graduate study.	American Speech and Hearing Association, 9030 Old Georgetown Rd., Washington, D.C., 20014.

GLOSSARY

Definitions of terms not included in the glossary may be found by consulting the index for text references.

analgesic
A drug that relieves pain.

anesthesiology
The science of anesthesia (the partial or complete loss of sensation with or without loss of consciousness resulting from the administration of drugs).

antihistamine
A drug which counters the effect on the body of naturally produced histamines; used to dry up the mucous membranes in the nose.

antiperspirant
A substance which works against both body odor and wetness.

apocrine glands
Sweat glands producing milky liquid which is decomposed by bacteria on the skin, producing body odor; has no known function.

bacterial plaques
Organized clusters of colonies of bacteria that inhabit the gumline of a tooth, which if not removed, cause decay, diseased gums, and foul breath.

cash indemnity
A cash benefit paid by a health insurance policy for an insured loss.

caveat emptor
Latin phrase meaning "let the buyer beware."

chiropractic
A system of therapy based upon the claim that disease is caused by abnormal function of the nervous system.

clinical psychologist One trained in the science of psychology who diagnoses and treats emotional and neurological conditions by the use of verbal and nonverbal methods.

comprehensive insurance A policy designed to give the protection offered by both a basic and major medical health insurance policy.

congenital Present at birth.

Consumer Price Index A government (U.S. Department of Labor) index for measuring changes in prices of consumer items, using prices of a given beginning (base) year as a comparison.

contact lenses Small plastic lenses that ride on a thin layer of tears directly over the cornea and under the eyelids.

coronary occlusion An obstruction in a branch of a coronary (heart) artery which hinders the flow of blood to some part of the heart muscle.

cosmetics Substances or articles applied to the body for cleansing, beautifying, promoting attractiveness, or altering appearance.

counsellor A psychologist advising people with normal problems.

debilitation Condition of weakness in functions or organs of the body.

deductible That portion of covered hospital and medical charges which an insured person must pay before his policy's benefits begin.

deodorant A substance which works against body odor.

dermatology The branch of medicine dealing with diagnosis and treatment of diseases of the skin.

diplomate A holder of a certificate of the National Board of Medical Examiners or of one of the American Boards of the Specialties; a *bona fide* specialist.

drug A substance which effects or alters normal body functioning.

eccrine glands Sweat glands producing clear odorless liquid to prevent the body from overheating.

elderly	A person aged 65 and older.
exclusions	Specified hazards for which a policy will not provide benefit payments.
family practice	The medical specialty concerned with the usual medical problems of a family unit, rather than with a particular body system or disease.
FDA	Food and Drug Administration; a federal regulatory agency concerned with consumer protection.
FTC	Federal Trade Commission; a federal regulatory agency concerned with unfair methods of competition in commerce.
general practitioner	One who practices the general, largely unrestricted, profession of medicine.
gynecology	The study of the diseases of the female, particularly of the genital, urinary, or rectal organs.
insuring clause	The clause which indicates the parties to a health insurance contract and states what is covered by the policy.
internal medicine	That department of medicine which deals with diseases that cannot be treated surgically.
internist	One who treats internal organs and diseases (not a surgeon) and who frequently confines his practice to adults.
JCAH	Joint Commission for the Accreditation of Hospitals; a national hospital accreditation organization.
medicare	A government program of health insurance under Social Security which helps the elderly pay for medical care.
mortality	A term used for death.
neurology	That branch of medicine dealing with the nervous system and its diseases.
noncancelable	A policy which the insured has the right to continue in force by the timely payment of premiums set forth in the policy to a specified age, during which period the insurer has no right to make, unilaterally, any

	change in any provision of the policy while the policy is in force.
nostrum	A medicine recommended by its preparer; a quack remedy; a cure-all.
nutrition labelling	Nutrient content in food labelling now required by the FDA.
obstetrics	That branch of medicine which deals with the care and treatment of women during pregnancy, childbirth, and the period immediately after.
ophthalmology	The branch of medicine dealing with the eye and its diseases.
osteopathy	A system of treating ailments which includes the belief that they generally result from the pressure of displaced bones on nerves, and are cured by manipulation.
otorhinolaryngology	The branch of medicine dealing with the ear, nose, and larynx and their functions and diseases.
paramedical	Having a medical aspect, or secondary relation to medicine.
patent medicine	A nonprescription medicine advertised to the public; often of secret composition.
pathology	That branch of medicine dealing with the nature of disease, especially the structural and functional changes caused by disease.
pediatrics	That branch of medicine which treats the development and care of children and the diseases of children and their treatment.
physician	A person authorized by law to practice medicine.
postnatal	Following birth.
pre-existing condition	A physical condition of an insured person which existed prior to the issuance of his policy.
premium	A periodic payment required to keep a policy in force.
proctology	The branch of medicine dealing with the rectum and its diseases.

proprietary   For the purpose of making a profit.

proprietary compound   A preparation for the treatment of disease, protected against free competition as to name, composition, or manufacturing process by secrecy, patent, copyright, trademark, or other means.

pseudo-science   False science.

psychiatry   That branch of medicine which deals with the diagnosis, treatment, and prevention of mental (emotional) illness.

psychologist   One trained in the science of psychology, that is, the study of the mind and behavior. They may engage in experimental, teaching, or clinical work.

quack   A boastful pretender to medical skill.

radiology   The branch of medicine which deals with roentgen rays and other radiant energy in the diagnosis and treatment of disease.

specialist   A practitioner who restricts himself to a special type of disease.

State Board Examination   A state examination in the medical, dental, or paramedical professions given by a State Board of Examiners from that particular profession, which, if passed, qualifies a person to practice that profession in that particular state.

surgery   The branch of medicine which treats diseases, partially or completely, by manual and operative procedures.

sympathomimetic   A drug which produces effects resembling those resulting from the stimulation of the sympathetic nervous system; used as nasal decongestants.

urology   That branch of medicine dealing with the urine and urinary tract.

waiting period   The duration of time between the beginning of an insured person's disability and the start of the policy's benefits.

SUPPLEMENTARY READING

American Cancer Society, *Volunteer* 16: 2 (1970).

American Medical Association, Council on Medical Service, *A Buyer's Guide to Health Insurance*. Chicago.

American Medical Association, *The Profile of Medical Practice, Reference Data on, 1972 Edition*. Chicago: 1972.

"An Overview of Cosmetics Regulation," *FDA Consumer* 6:3 (April 1972).

"A Revolution in Cosmetics Regulation," *FDA Consumer* 8:3 (April 1974).

Blue Cross Association and National Association of Blue Shield Plans, *Blue Cross and Blue Shield Fact Book, 1974*. Chicago: 1974.

Bock, William B., and Sperberg, Mary J., *Directory of Prepaid Dental Care Plans, 1967*. Bethesda: U.S. Department of Health, Education, and Welfare, 1968.

"Can Your Kitchen Pass the Food Storage Test?," *FDA Consumer* 8:2 (March 1974).

Crichton, Michael, "The High Cost of Cure," *Atlanta* 225:3 (March 1970).

"Drug Pricing and the Rx Police State," *Consumer Reports* 37:3 (March 1972).

Editors of Consumer Reports, *The Medicine Show*. Mount Vernon: 1963.

"Eye Products: Handle with Care," *FDA Consumer* 6:6 (July-August 1972).

"FDA Annual Report, 1971," Special Edition, *FDA Consumer* 5:10 (December 1971-January 1972).

Health Insurance Institute, *Source Book of Health Insurance Data, 1973–74*. New York: 1974.

Jones, Kenneth L., Shainberg, Louis W., and Byer, Curtis O., *Dimensions, A Changing Concept of Health.* San Francisco: Canfield Press, 1974.

Jones, Kenneth L., Shainberg, Louis W., and Byer, Curtis O., *Health Science.* New York: Harper and Row, 1974.

Katz, Sol, "Evaluating Cold Remedies," *Today's Health* 48:6 (June 1970).

Kime, Robert E., Health: *A Consumer's Dilemma.* Belmont: Wadsworth Publishing Company, 1970.

Marmelstein, Neil, "Sweat Is Almost Obsolete," *Today's Health* 48:6 (June 1970).

"Myths of Vitamins," *FDA Consumer* 8:2 (March 1974).

National Academy of Sciences, National Research Council, Food and Nutrition Board, *Recommended Dietary Allowances, 8th Edition.* Washington: 1973.

"Nutrition Labels: A Great Leap Forward," *FDA Consumer* 7:7 (September 1973).

Ochsner, Alton, "Medical Breakthroughs You Can Expect in 10, 25, 50 Years," *Today's Health* 51:4 (April 1973).

"Prescription Drugs—The War Over Secret Prices," *Changing Times,* 27:2 (February 1973).

"Reducing Injuries From Shattered Eyeglasses," *FDA Consumer* 6:6 (March 1972).

"$60 Billion Crisis Over Medical Care," *Business Week* 2107 (January 17, 1970).

"Sun Worship," *Today's Health* 48:6 (June 1970).

"The Hexachlorophene Story," *FDA Consumer* 6:3 (April 1972).

U.S. Department of Agriculture, *Food For Us All, The Yearbook of Agriculture, 1969.* Washington: 1969.

U.S. Department of Health, Education, and Welfare, *Health Manpower Source Book, Section 21, Allied Health Manpower, 1950–80.* Washington: Public Health Service, National Institutes of Health, Publication No. 263, 1970.

U.S. Department of Health, Education, and Welfare, *Health Resources Statistics, Health Manpower,* and *Health Facilities, 1972–73.* Washington: Public Health Service, Publication No. (HSM) 73-1509, 1973.

U.S. Department of Health, Education, and Welfare, *Vital Statistics of the U.S.* Washington: Public Health Service, 1974.

U.S. Department of Labor, *Occupational Outlook Handbook, 1974–75 Edition.* Washington: 1974.

"Vitamin E—Miracle or Myth," *FDA Consumer* 7:6 (July-August 1973).

INDEX

Italic page numbers indicate that reference will be found in a table or figure.